Routledge Revivals

The Clinical Experience

This second edition, published in 1991 follows the original edition from 1981 which was the only published ethnography of medical education in the UK. The theoretical, methodological and substantive issues continue to be of importance to the sociology and anthropology of medicine and medical knowledge. Indeed, critiques of contemporary 'biomedicine' and the growing interest in the sociology of the body have made its central concerns of even greater significance than when the first edition was published.

Covering topics including the clinical tradition, the social distribution of bedside knowledge, reproducing disease, and the clinical setting, this expanded edition builds on the success of the first and will interest researchers and clinicians in the fields of sociology, anthropology and medicine.

This book was originally published as part of the *Cardiff Papers in Qualitative Research* series edited by Paul Atkinson, Sara Delamont and Amanda Coffey. The series publishes original sociological research that reflects the tradition of qualitative and ethnographic inquiry developed at Cardiff. The series includes monographs reporting on empirical research, edited collections focussing on particular themes, and texts discussing methodological developments and issues.

The Clinical Experience
The Construction and Reconstruction of Medical Reality
Second Edition

Paul Atkinson

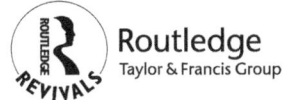

Routledge
Taylor & Francis Group

First published in 1997
by Avebury, Ashgate Publishing Limited

This edition first published in 2018 by Routledge
2 Park Square, Milton Park, Abingdon, Oxon, OX14 4RN
and by Routledge
711 Third Avenue, New York, NY 10017

Routledge is an imprint of the Taylor & Francis Group, an informa business

© 1997 Paul Atkinson

Publisher's Note
The publisher has gone to great lengths to ensure the quality of this reprint but points out that some imperfections in the original copies may be apparent.

Disclaimer
The publisher has made every effort to trace copyright holders and welcomes correspondence from those they have been unable to contact.

A Library of Congress record exists under LCCN: 97073874

ISBN 13: 978-0-8153-8470-0 (hbk)
ISBN 13: 978-1-351-20355-5 (ebk)
ISBN 13: 978-0-8153-8471-7 (pbk)

The Clinical Experience

The construction and reconstruction of medical reality

Second edition

PAUL ATKINSON
School of Social and Administrative Studies
University of Wales, Cardiff

Ashgate

Aldershot • Brookfield USA • Singapore • Sydney

Published by
Ashgate Publishing Ltd
Gower House
Croft Road
Aldershot
Hants GU11 3HR
England

Ashgate Publishing Company
Old Post Road
Brookfield
Vermont 05036
USA

British Library Cataloguing in Publication Data

Atkinson, Paul
   The clinical experience : the construction and
   reconstruction of medical reality. - 2nd ed. -(Cardiff
   papers in qualitative research)
   1. Social medicine 2. Clinical medicine - Social aspects
   I. Title
   306.4'61

Library of Congress Catalog Card Number: 97-73874

ISBN 1 85628 577 4

Contents

Preface to the second edition

There are several reasons why I have brought out a second edition of this monograph. It has, of course, given me the opportunity to expand upon and improve (I hope) on the presentation of the empirical material contained in the first edition of 1981. There are issues that were contained in the original ethnography that for one reason or another did not feature in the first edition. It was a severely pruned version of my PhD thesis, and in the necessary editorial work that went into the production of a short monograph some material was lost that, in retrospect, might well have been included. In particular, for historical reasons that I have alluded to elsewhere (Atkinson 1992), the original doctoral thesis and the resulting monograph both under-reported work I carried out in observing the teaching of surgery. I concentrated most of my writing on the teaching of general medicine, despite having spent almost as long observing in surgical settings. This second edition has allowed me to go some way towards redressing the balance, and of introducing a modest amount of material that was previously unpublished.

Furthermore, the subject-matter of my original research still remains rather neglected in British sociology of medicine and of the professions. The social processes whereby medical work and medical knowledge are reproduced remain poorly documented. Whether or not one's academic colleagues believe (mistakenly) that is has 'been done', or that the subject is lacking in intrinsic interest, the fact remains that there has been little published in the vein of *The Clinical Experience* in the years since its first appearance. This is so despite the fact that recent developments in the sociology and anthropology of medical knowledge place such interests at the heart of the discipline. Since the original monograph has long been out of print, and the original edition ran to a short print run only, it seems to me that it is not only personal hubris that commends a new edition that may bring these issues to a new and wider readership.

In revising and expanding this edition, I have taken some general decisions on how to proceed. The data themselves are undeniably old, having been collected in the early 1970s, and partially published from then onwards. I have not pretended that the empirical materials are current: I have not tried to up-date the details of medical education in order to create the appearance of contemporary work in that substantive sense. I do not imagine, nor do I intend to imply, that medical education in Britain or elsewhere is timeless. On the other hand, I think that there is good reason to believe - as I discuss more fully in what follows - that many of the fundamental rituals and routines of clinical instruction have changed rather slowly. Indeed, there seems to be a massive cultural inertia that preserves and cherishes many of the features described here and in similar works. On the other hand, I have resisted the possibility of changing the entire monograph into the past tense. I have decided to maintain the use of the 'ethnographic present'. I am aware of the dangers that such a textual practice entails. Its ideological and epistemological consequences have been explored by others (e.g. Fabian 1983). This practice, long associated with ethnographic writing in sociology and anthropology, can too readily convey the impression of a social world that is 'out of time'. As I have suggested myself (Atkinson 1992) it is all too easy for the ethnographic monograph to collapse the concrete social action it reports into a kind of dream-time that mythologizes its subject-matter. On the other hand, the ethnographic present serves to reinforce the immediacy of the original ethnographic work. It recreates, sometimes vividly, the social scenes, actors and activities in a way that the distance of the past tense can never allow. Consequently I have allowed myself to retain the original, and well established usage of the present tense.

Equally, I have not attempted to re-write the ethnography as if all the contemporary literature and theories were available to me in 1976 when I completed the doctoral thesis, or in 1981 when the first edition of this monograph was published. I have tried to indicate at various key points how this ethnography relates to key ideas and themes in the sociology of medicine, of the body and so on. But I have not grafted the equivalent of an anachronistic review of the literature onto the original work. To a considerable extent, therefore, the work retains most of its original features. I have, however, exercised self-indulgence in one particular area. Since completing the research and the monograph, I have had the opportunity to contribute to general methodological literature on the conduct of ethnography, and have published on the conduct of this particular field project. In the original version, an extended account of the research methods was one major casualty of the editorial transformation

vii

of thesis into monograph. I have therefore taken the liberty of reinstating a more extended account of the conduct of the research. By analogy with several other ethnographies, then, this may be thought of as the 'fieldwork edition' of *The Clinical Experience*.

For their help in preparing this edition I am grateful to Laura Pugsley, Elizabeth Renton and Jackie Swift. I am also grateful to Sara Delamont and Amanda Coffey, who helped to establish the Cardiff Papers series, for their support and encouragement.

1 The clinical tradition

Introduction

The setting is a hospital ward of unmistakably nineteenth century origins. In a large open ward a number of patients are sitting up in bed, more or less comfortable. Nurses are bustling about, dressed in a bewildering variety of colours and styles of uniform. There are several other workers coming in and out of the ward. A portable X-ray machine is wheeled in, and a patient is wheeled out. A physiotherapist is looking for her patient, who seems to have disappeared; the therapist acknowledges defeat and leaves. The furniture and equipment on the ward is modern, but shabby and looks uncared for. The paintwork manages to be simultaneously fresh and drab. There is little here to invoke the wonders of modern high technology medicine, nor yet to provoke anxiety. There is no drama, no heroics. The patients appear listless, preoccupied with their own solitude rather than suffering.

Into this ward comes a small group of men and women, all wearing white coats. Most of them are in their early twenties. An older man is clearly in charge. Whereas the youngsters seem unsure of themselves, he enters the ward with an easy air of self assurance. He radiates authority. They group together at the door and mutter together conspiratorially, occasionally throwing glances at the occupant of a bed. The patients and the staff take little notice of the intrusion. Most of them are well used to these incursions. We are in a teaching hospital, and a teaching 'round' is in progress. A consultant physician is taking a small group of medical students to talk to and examine one or more of his patients in the ward.

The huddle breaks up, and the physician and his students make their way towards one particular bed. They form themselves into a new group round the patient; the consultant stands at the head of the bed, to the patient's right and the students range below him on both sides of the bed. The screens are pulled round the huddle, and the patient is entirely hidden behind curtains and bodies. The patient herself is a skinny woman, with coarse, iron grey hair and a sallow complexion. The consultant introduces her to the students. She is sixty-two years old, and has been complaining of breathlessness, but she displays no other signs of distress, nor does she seem to be discomfited by the arrival of the doctor and his students.

The consultant turns to one of the students and asks him to start examining the patient:

> 'What system would you want to examine in relation to Mrs. Baxter's breathlessness?'
>
> 'The cardiovascular system ... and the respiratory', the student replies.
>
> 'What about anaemia?'
>
> 'I was including that in the cardiovascular, 'cos blood goes through that ...'

The other students and the doctor chuckle at this apparent gaffe, while its perpetrator looks ashamed and embarrassed. He then begins to examine the patient. Meanwhile a couple of the other students have picked up the patient's chart which is hanging at the foot of the bed. The consultant spots them and they are scolded, 'You'll be able to tell what's wrong with her just by looking at the treatment she's getting'. And so the teaching continues. The students take turns at examining the patient, questioning her and responding to questions from the doctor. The patient replies when she is spoken to, but otherwise takes no active part in the proceedings. She is a compliant lay figure.

That brief description of a round in an Edinburgh teaching hospital would, I assume, come as no great surprise to anyone. Even if it is not something one had experienced, from one or other side of the bedclothes, it is part and parcel of our stock of knowledge of how doctors are trained. It is an archetype, just like the family doctor taking a pulse, or the school teacher lecturing in front of a blackboard.

It is this archetype which forms the theme of this monograph, which is addressed to the clinical elements in undergraduate medical education. It is based on a two-year period of participant observation in the Edinburgh medical school, when I observed bedside teaching in medicine and surgery during the students' first year of clinical studies. What is presented in this book is a highly selective account of just one aspect of that ethnographic study: the social construction and reconstruction of medical reality (cf. Berger and Luckmann, 1967; Atkinson, 1977).

I have no intention of attempting to produce a comprehensive account of the socialisation process, of how medical students become doctors. My research was not a longitudinal study of cohorts of students, and in any event the notion of socialisation is highly problematic in this context (Olesen and Whittaker, 1970; Dingwall, 1977). Rather, I concentrate on one particular, crucial phase within the undergraduate course at one medical school. That is, the students' initial exposure to the 'reality' of clinical medicine.

The clinical experience

Doctors' own reminiscences of their student days are full of vividly drawn accounts of their initial encounters with the mysteries of clinical medicine, and the awesome, theatrical, quirky or otherwise remarkable people who were responsible for their initiation. Those early, hesitant steps in clinical medicine mark a major turning-point in any doctor's individual, professional biography. It is part of the stock of personal mythology by which a doctor can trace out some of the salient features of his or her identity as a medical practitioner. Remembered with a mixture of fondness, pride and horror, these portraits of the past are familiar. They have been accurately lampooned by Ferris (1967): 'I well remember Sir Egbert telling me "always examine the patient in an easterly light".'

This is the very stuff of personal medical mythology. It also serves to establish a collective, shared 'mythological charter'. For the clinical tradition is central to the culture of medicine, and to the transmission of that culture. Bedside medicine and bedside teaching, together with the knowledge that is produced and reproduced at the bedside, are granted a privileged status in the clinical tradition. Foucault (1973) has suggested that it is fundamental to the self-definition of modern medicine. As Foucault describes it, the clinic is taken to provide the rationale for medicine's characteristic empiricism, and the priority granted to personal experience and firsthand perception at the patient's bedside:

> Medicine has tended, since the eighteenth century, to recount its own history as if the patient's bedside had always been a place of constant, stable experience, in contrast to theories and systems which had been in perpetual change and masked beneath their speculation the purity of clinical evidence. (p.54)

The clinic, whose birth Foucault uncovers, was the distinctive combination of new investigative technology, the reorganisation of medical discourse, the rise of the great teaching hospitals and so on. This conjuncture, he argues, produced a characteristic and revolutionary mode of perception and understanding. Whereas previous theorising had allowed for the natural history and classification of disease (often in the most elaborate nosologies), the clinic was born when it became permissible to treat the individual as a field of medical-clinical-investigation: 'one could at last hold a scientifically structured discourse about an individual'. The space of the patient's bedside thus became a new locus of inquiry and research as well as treatment and instruction.

In this clinical space, the doctor's own direct scrutiny of the patient became invested with a new significance. Under the hospital physician's gaze (*le regard*) the superstructure of theory fell away to reveal a pure, uncontaminated perception of the patient and his illness. Or such became the mythological charter:

> Clinical experience ... was soon taken as a simple, unconceptualized confrontation of a gaze and a face, or a glance and a silent body; a sort of contact prior to all discourse, free of all the burdens of language, by which two living individuals are 'trapped' in a common, but non-reciprocal situation. (Foucault, 1973, p.xiv)

Foucault, of course, is arguing a very particular thesis concerning the emergence of a novel system of thought and practice in revolutionary and post-revolutionary France. In doing so he almost certainly over emphasises the extent to which there was a radical break with the medical past. The clinical gaze was granted a new and enhanced status, but the clinical tradition and its mythology extends back beyond the moment of its birth that Foucault identifies.

Any search for absolute origins is bound to fail, and it is in the very nature of mythological charters that their remoter periods are subject to change. Early generations are confused and compressed; the relation to cult figures and heroes does not necessarily correspond to the niceties of historical accuracy. But the figure of Boerhaave is noteworthy in the development of eighteenth-century clinical work. Foremost among the theorists and teachers at Leyden, Boerhaave's influence was profound and widespread. Appositely for this book, it was Boerhaave who provided the major influence on the early days of the medical school at Edinburgh. The medical school itself was established on the Continental model, and several of the early teachers were trained at Leyden, which was then the foremost centre of medical theory, practice and instruction (Comrie, 1932).

The practice of bedside teaching at Edinburgh, based on the Leyden model, was recognisably the predecessor of later approaches to clinical instruction, such as those Foucault describes:

> The Chief would go round the ward with his student and coming to the bed the Chief would stand at the top of the bed and the student would stand by the patient. The Chief would ask the student a question, the student would then speak to the patient, the patient would reply to the student, the student would shout at the top of his voice the answer to the assembled students and the Chief would hear the answer.
>
> (Eastwood, 1972)

In the eighteenth century, at medical schools like Leyden and Edinburgh, the clinical tradition was established. This 'old clinic' was a medicine of symptoms: there was little or no investigation of the patient's body for signs of pathology:

> The actual methods of teaching students were much the same in 1800 as they are today, with one great exception, the development of the technique of teaching due to that revolution in the technique of Medicine, the invention of the physical examination of the patient. This innovation demanded the introduction of methods of teaching the elicitation of physical signs, and the provision of those opportunities for practice and experience on which this interpretation and evaluation must be based.
>
> (Newman, 1957, p.30)

The clinical tradition established by Boerhaave's followers and others in the eighteenth century, then, coupled with the new technology and emergent specialties of the nineteenth century, provides the basis for this mythological charter for medicine and its distinctive cultural reproduction. The emergence of the clinic and its special status in the tradition of modern medicine has also been noted by Jamous and Peloille (1970). Their argument has many points of contact with Foucault's version. They describe how, during the early years of the last century, the roles of teacher, researcher and clinician became fused in the University hospitals in France. The hospital wards were the main research environment, as well as a locale for training and patient care. But as the century went on, this conjunction was threatened and fragmented. With the emergence of the laboratory based research (such as bacteriology), the clinician lost his monopoly over the production and use of medical knowledge. Within the medical profession, Jamous and Peloille argue, there emerged a struggle for supremacy between the clinicians and the non clinical scientists.

The detail of Jamous and Peloille's argument does not concern us here. They do, however, draw attention to the most important point. They document how hospital clinicians attempted to reassert their superiority by means of appeals to their own pre-theoretical clinical experience. By virtue of their clinical gaze the clinicians laid claim to a privileged perception. This arcane knowledge and experience was, it was claimed, 'indeterminate', in contrast to the 'technical' rationality of the scientific disciplines. In their own discussion of actual historical events, Jamous and Peloille are guilty of reifying their notion of technicality and indetermination and of over-simplifying the historical relationships between competing definitions of medical knowledge. None the less, they are right to point out the centrality of knowledge which is defined as indeterminate. That is, knowledge which practitioners believe is not susceptible to rational codification and explicit statement. All crafts and occupations have such areas (though the boundaries of technicality and indetermination will often be disputed by members of occupational groups).

In the context of medicine, such indeterminate knowledge has been associated with the notion of clinical experience. It has been vouchsafed by the privilege of the clinical gaze. This in turn has guaranteed the centrality of bedside teaching as the mode of cultural transmission whereby such knowledge may be imparted. It depends upon the novice, or apprentice, being exposed directly to the signs and symptoms of illness. Despite the fragmentation of medical knowledge and teaching, the growth of new specialties and the increasing importance of science and technology, the clinic and bedside teaching have retained a central importance. Throughout the changes in theory and practice of medical education, the clinical - and its transmission through bedside teaching - has remained, in its essentials, unaltered. Its justification remains that which Foucault and Jamous and Peloille identify from earlier epochs - an appeal to direct, pre-theoretical experience and the accumulation of personal, clinical experience.

If the clinic was born in the period described by Foucault, or in yet earlier years, then it is re-born every day. It enjoys a daily renaissance in the ward rounds of contemporary clinicians and their students. In the training of medical students, individual biographies and the collective tradition of the medical profession flow together. Here too are fused the components of theory and practice, science and practical experience.

Clinical experience and the lessons of the bedside are central to the past and the present of clinical culture. Such a distinctive organisation of knowledge and perception gives rise to what Freidson (1970) described as the *clinical mentality*. Freidson distinguishes the medical practitioner, the clinician, from the theorist or the scientist. The clinician's primary orientation is towards *action* - so much so that he or she may prefer to do something with very uncertain chances of success over taking no action at all. The practitioner, Freidson argues, 'believes in what he [sic] is doing'. That is, the clinician is likely to display a personal commitment to his or her chosen course of action. The practitioner is essentially a pragmatist, relying on results rather than theory, and trusting in personal, firsthand knowledge rather than on abstract principles or 'book knowledge'.

These components, all mutually interdependent, comprise a distinctive occupational culture, characterised by a particular orientation towards knowledge and action. The clinical approach comes to induce in the practitioner an ultimate trust in the evidence of his or her senses, and the warrant of his or her personal knowledge or experience. This Freidson summarises as 'a rather thoroughgoing particularism, a kind of ontological and epistemological individualism'. It is the warrant for individual action, and the competence of a practitioner may be judged (by colleagues, for instance) by reference to the essentially biographical notion of personal experience.

Freidson's remarks on the clinical mentality are drawn in part from Becker *et al.* (1961). In their study of medical students at Kansas they noted the importance of the 'experience perspective' in organising the views of staff and students. They summarise the perspective in this way:

> It is important for a doctor to have had clinical experience
> .... School activities are good insofar as they give students
> the opportunity to acquire clinical experience or give them
> access to the clinical experience of their teachers; they are
> bad when they furnish neither of these things .... A student
> is making real progress towards his goal of preparing for
> practice when he can demonstrate to himself and others
> that he has absorbed some lessons from clinical experience;

conversely, he has cause to be worried over his own
abilities when he fails to absorb such lessons. (p.242)

Although it is not the only available criterion, the notion of clinical
experience is often used as a touchstone in the evaluation of some course
of action, or in choosing between competing approaches. As Becker and
his co-authors go on to comment, 'actual experience in dealing with
patients and disease' is often used in contrast to 'theoretical' and
'scientific' knowledge:

> ... even though it substitutes for scientifically verified
> knowledge, it can be used to legitimate a choice of
> procedures for a patient's treatment and can even be used
> to rule out use of some procedures that have been
> scientifically established. (p.225)

In this context, 'scientifically established' should not be understood in any
absolute sense. What is at issue is what *passes* for up-to-date, validated
scientific procedure - incorporated in research papers, learned journals,
textbooks and so on. Scientific knowledge and personal experience are
equally social in their definition, but the warrants claimed for them are
different. The clinical culture is predicated, therefore, on the personal
accumulation of clinical experience, and such a stock of knowledge is an
essential component of any practitioner's competence. It is acquired in
large measure at the patient's bedside - that personal and perceptual space
encompassed by the clinical gaze.

Historically speaking the apprenticeship model of medical training has
become somewhat attenuated. The attachment of a young novice doctor to
the firm of a mentor no longer plays the part it once did, and is but one of
a wide range of educational experiences the medical student is exposed to.
Similarly, the student's actual responsibility for the day-to-day care of the
patient has been postponed. The junior student is no longer, as Flexner
(1925) described, 'part of the functioning machine'. Junior medical
students in their early days of clinical medicine or surgery are much less
frequently expected to undertake the routine and menial tasks once
expected of a clerk or dresser.

Nonetheless, the underlying mode of teaching and learning retains
core features of apprenticeship. Though junior students do not play an
important part in the daily work of the ward, they still gain their clinical
understanding through exposure to the world of the hospital. Students are
expected to acquire their expertise, and to accumulate their store of

experience, largely from the example of their clinical teachers. They learn by example: by observing at the bedside, in the clinic, from the gallery or on the floor of the operating theatre. They acquire their competence through supervised practical work, in the 'real-life' context of medical practice. Even though their diagnoses and opinions are not actually implemented and do not normally affect the management of patients, students are called upon to examine, diagnose and recommend treatment *as if* they were indeed responsible for the patients they encounter. Although they are not usually entrusted with work of real importance, junior students learn 'on the job'.

In the transmission of the clinical culture, its enactment in bedside teaching is of fundamental importance. But despite its centrality to medical education and its mythological significance, bedside teaching has remained almost entirely neglected as a topic of sociological research.

The invisible clinic

Medical students are often used as a benchmark in the literature on professional socialisation, as well as in the sociology of medicine. The place of medical education has been secured in the sociological literature by two classic studies. The first was based upon the teaching programme at Cornell, and was undertaken by members of the Columbia University Bureau of Applied Social Research (Merton *et al.*, 1957). The second, a study of Kansas University medical school was done by members of a research group in sociology at the University of Chicago (Becker *et al.*, 1961). The contrasting portrayals of medical education and student life offered by these two studies have become reference points in the literature on professional socialisation.

Arguably, the undoubted quality and importance of the two classics has had an inhibiting effect on subsequent researchers, both in Britain and elsewhere. There seems to have been a willingness on the part of many British sociologists to believe that medical education has been 'done', and to rely almost exclusively on the American sources. Elsewhere, notably in the United States, subsequent research has been undertaken. But the inhibitory effect of the early studies is apparent. There is a tendency for later research almost obsessively to recapitulate the problems and perspectives laid down by the Columbia and Chicago studies. It is not my intention to review this debate in any detail, but a brief summary is unavoidable.

While they have been fascinated by the professions for many years, sociologists have, while claiming to demystify them, been mystified in their turn (cf. Roth, 1974). Sociological observers of the professions have repeatedly found themselves entangled in a web of definitional problems. Indeed, the very meanings of the term 'professions' and 'professional' have proved a stumbling block, and their value as sociological concepts has been much contested.

In simple terms one can identify two competing approaches: one which seeks to identify 'professions' as distinctive, special sorts of occupations, and one which denies any inherent qualities which might set them apart. The first approach takes as a dominant theme the identification of the *differentia specifica* of the professions. In some of their characteristic forms such approaches are referred to as 'trait' theories. The task of delineating a distinctive category of 'professions' has proved troublesome. Many of the proposed lists have proved incompatible; while all or some of the traits appear to apply to so-called professions, they apply also to occupations not so designated; often it is far from clear where the traits are derived from. Many of the characteristics appear to have been incorporated from the occupations' public self presentation and 'bootlegged' into the sociologists' definitions.

The second approach avoids such pitfalls. It derives in large measure from the work of Everett Hughes (1958). The crucial question, it is maintained, is not 'what is a profession?' but rather 'when do people begin to apply this label to themselves?' In other words, 'profession' and 'professional' are self designations or claims made for and by particular occupational groups. There is, according to this view, nothing inherent in the work, training, or personnel which denotes 'professions' as a particular class of occupation.

The first approach, associated with functionalist theorising, coloured the research of the Columbia group, and their account of medical education. The latter, distinctly interactionist perspective, underlies the work of the Chicago school. Merton and his collaborators have in mind a distinctive set of roles and values as the *terminus ad quem* of training. Medical students are:

> engaged in learning the professional role of the physician
> by so combining its component knowledge and skills,
> attitudes and values, as to be motivated and able to perform
> their role in a professionally and socially acceptable
> fashion. (p.41)

In this view the distinctive knowledge, attitudes and values of the fully-fledged professional are seen as being laid down during the initial training period.

Becker and his colleagues, on the other hand, stress the immediate, day-to-day experience of medical school life, and play down the relationship between basic education and future performance as a competent practitioner. Rather than assuming the assimilation of a repertoire of roles and values, the Chicago researchers concentrate on how students survive and they get through medical school.

The two approaches can be seen as attempts, more or less successful, to answer two different questions. The Columbia study asked, 'How do people become doctors?' The emphasis of the Chicago study was rather focused on 'learning the ropes': initiates are faced with immediate, practical problems of 'getting by' in novel situations and must find ways of coping. Miller (1970, p.118) summarises this approach:

> Newcomers in any social situation go through an initial process of learning the ropes: finding out who the other people in that situation are, where they are located, what they do, what they expect the newcomer to do, and how they want him to do it. We seldom dignify this process by calling it learning.

Yet it is precisely this aspect of 'learning' that is seized on by Becker and his co-workers.

In line with these differing perspectives, too, the two studies portray student life in very different terms - aptly caught in their respective titles. The 'student physician' is described as a junior partner in the training process, who is sponsored toward full membership of the profession by his teachers. The 'boy in white' is seen as occupying a much more lowly position, and enjoying very different relationships with medical school staff. There is a strong social barrier between the staff and students and a divergence between their respective preoccupations and interests. Each study describes a 'student culture', but ascribes very different characteristics to them. The Columbia research describes student culture as comprising a 'little society' in which the professional norms of the faculty are reflected and reinforced. At Kansas, the student culture appears almost to be an 'underground resistance movement', in which students unite against a hostile and threatening environment.

These two positions, to a considerable extent, have provided taken for granted reference points, either in terms of guiding subsequent work, or inhibiting more original approaches. But they do not represent the only possible perspectives. Neither their subject matter nor their approaches to medical education is exhaustive. There have been major *lacunae* in their coverage (and in subsequently published research projects). In particular both the Columbia study and the Chicago-school research at Kansas neglected the topic of clinical teaching. Merton and his colleagues focus on students' attitudes towards medicine and types of patients, but remain silent on the nature of the student-patient encounter. Likewise, Becker and his co-authors remark on students' attitudes; but 'Students and Patients' is given only brief attention, and 'Student-Patient Interaction' occupies a bare two pages in what is a lengthy monograph. More recent studies of medical education have also tended to gloss over the particular topic of clinical, bedside instruction.

Perhaps the most disappointing of all these omissions was that of the Chicago school. The authors note that 'The student spends much of his [sic] time in the clinical years interacting with patients', yet they offer only a brief and idealised description of the student-patient encounter:

> The third year student typically meets his patients when they are hospitalised for diagnosis and treatment. He comes into contact with them repeatedly during their hospital stay. He performs a complete examination upon the patient's arrival in the hospital. He presents the patient to the staff and other students during the rounds, describing the case in detail, demonstrating outstanding clinical findings, and suggesting a diagnosis and plan of treatment. He checks daily on the patient's progress, quizzing and re-examining the patient frequently. He enters into a casual but continuing relationship with the patient. The major problem patients present for the student on the hospital wards, then, is to maintain this continuing relationship in such a fashion as to be able to get the necessary information he is assigned. (p.315)

In this highly compressed account Becker and his colleagues gloss over a wide range of skills, problems and social encounters: students must engage in purposeful talk with patients, perform examinations, formulate histories and generate diagnoses. Students must generate displays of ability, under the scrutiny of their clinical teachers, and present a 'front' of competence. Through the focused encounters of bedside interaction, medical knowledge is transmitted in a dramatic fashion. Yet all this has remained strangely neglected. Bedside teaching has remained largely unexamined from within medicine. While medical school members have themselves engaged vigorously in research and innovation, they have tended to concentrate on such topics as methods of selection and assessment, career choice, psychological assessment and so on. One author (Crooks, 1974) has been moved to describe the topic of bedside clinical instruction as 'taboo'.

To some extent the state of research reflects dominant interests on the part of both sociological observers, and medical educators. But the neglect of bedside teaching may go rather deeper than that. It may lie in the nature of the enterprise itself and its taken-for-granted legitimacy, in that it apparently depends on the students' direct exposure to the 'reality' of medical work. Such firsthand experience may appear to need no further elaboration or justification. It can appear so 'obvious' and 'natural' that direct observation and investigation in turn appear unnecessary. Just as bedside work provides a traditional justification for the distinctive clinical culture, so it has a self-justificatory aim in its day to day accomplishment.

Bedside teaching may also have remained relatively invisible for another reason. Crooks' description of clinical instruction as 'taboo' seems particularly apt. There is more than a hint that bedside experience is regarded as the most sacred of the mysteries which only the initiated may be party to. Exposure to this world constitutes a core of the extended *rite de passage* of the medical student. Although there has been a considerable amount of curricular innovation in British medical schools in recent years, the centrality of clinical instruction in the major hospital subjects (primarily medicine and surgery) has remained. Introductory courses in clinical method tend to be focused on the classical concerns of history taking, physical examination and diagnostic inference on the wards of the teaching hospital. The clinic remains self-evidently at the heart of the clinical, and the clinic at the heart of medical training.

The clinical tradition is captured and re-enacted through the *spectacle of the clinic*. It is no mere accident of history that one of the most abiding images of the history of medicine is the distinctive medical lecture theatre - based on the Padua model. The steeply raked circle or oval in which students can look down on and observe an anatomical dissection or a living patient is in itself an icon of medical instruction. This theatre-in-the-round is not the only dramatic element in the oral tradition of medical culture. Clinical instruction is couched in an idiom of the spectacle. Contemporary practice retains the clinical presentation, for instance. Patients may be 'presented' to an audience of students in a lecture-theatre, in a ritualised form of display and recitation that recapitulates generations of clinical instruction. Likewise, the surgical operating *theatre* (and again, the dramaturgical metaphor is apt) provides a setting for the spectacular enactment of clinical work. With a gallery from which students and others can observe, and a running commentary conducted by the surgeon, the operating theatre physically embodies the clinical tradition: a collective gaze is focused on the patient's body, and on the person of the surgeon. The active surgeon or physician and the passive patient, surrounded by a group of witnesses, is also reproduced in the teaching rounds that form much of the substance of this book. The teaching physician or surgeon, followed by a retinue of students or others, takes on the role of *thaumaturge*, a wonder-working magus who displays and demonstrates his (more rarely, her) virtuosity. Before the audience of novices, the clinician manages displays of diagnostic insight and skilled technique. The signs and symptoms of disease are thus constituted as elements in a stage-managed spectacle. In several of the chapters that follow, I shall explore some of the key features of the clinical drama and its production.

In the years since the fieldwork for this monograph was completed, sociologists and anthropologists have paid increasing attention to the cultures of modern medicine. They have characterised it as a collection of beliefs and practices like any other cultural system: one ethnomedicine among many. The scrutiny of anthropological strangeness has often been shifted from the exotic systems of non-Western cultures in order to examine the medical rationalities of our own cultural practices. Equally, sociologists of health and illness have devoted increasing attention to the social construction of medical knowledge. Despite these intellectual trends, however, there has been a disappointing lack of interest in the processes of knowledge production and reproduction through medical curriculum and pedagogy. Equally, while the sociology of education has included a strand on the sociology of curricular knowledge, its focus has all too rarely strayed beyond the bounds of schooling. The reproduction of professional knowledge, including the practice of medical education, remains beyond the pale of the sociology of education. As a consequence there has been little published work that develops still further our sociological or anthropoological understanding of how medical knowledge is produced and reproduced in medical schools and teaching hospitals.

Postscript

Since the completion of my fieldwork and the publication of the first edition of this monograph, the overall pattern of medical education in the United Kingdom has changed. The changes have culminated in recommendations from the General Medical Council that finally and formally eliminate the division between clinical and preclinical phases. That divide, and the internal divisions between different subjects and specialties have been weakened. Vertical and horizontal integration have become the organising principles of medical curricula based on major thematic strands that span the entire period of undergraduate training. The emphasis is on problem-solving skills rather than the acquisition of large volumes of factual material. In many ways, therefore, medical education at the end of the century is organised on lines very different from those that informed the clinical instruction that I observed.

It is, however, too soon, and we have too little research to go on, to tell whether the pervasive culture of medicine has been transformed in accordance with the new approaches to curriculum and pedagogy. Indeed, it is part of the general background to this book that the forms of medical knowledge and medical instruction change slowly. There appear to be formal features of the culture that are highly resistant to profound transformation. If that argument is right, then we shall see the same reproduction of medical reality embedded in changing rhetorics of educational management. If that is right, as I strongly suspect, then the clinical gaze and the oral tradition will continue to be core elements in the medical mystique, and clinical experience will continue to occupy a privileged position in medical culture.

Although we lack published field research on change and persistence in British medical schools, anecdotal evidence continues to suggest that there is indeed innovation without change in this respect. Notwithstanding the transformations in policy and the corresponding adjustments to curriculum and delivery, it appears to be the case that 'traditional' clinical practice and clinical instruction retain their fundamental significance.

2 Entering the clinical world

The Royal Infirmary, the main teaching hospital at Edinburgh, stands next to the quadrangle of the Faculty of Medicine, which contains the laboratories, lecture theatres and library. The two are separated by a tree lined walk which leads into the Meadows, a large park. Student tradition has it that it is a matter of some moment whether, on arriving first thing in the morning, one turns to the east into the pre-clinical building, or westwards, into the Infirmary. The physical proximity of the two sets of buildings and their separation mirrors the divide between the two main phases of the undergraduate curriculum, and a decisive break in students' careers. The majority of students regard the transition from preclinical to clinical work as a particularly critical status passage in the course of their training. The undergraduate curriculum at Edinburgh follows the traditional pattern in dividing the course into these two major segments. The preclinical sequence spans a first-year (1st M.B.) phase of basic science and two subsequent years of preclinical science, including Anatomy, Physiology, Biochemistry, Pathology and Bacteriology. The majority of students enter directly to the second year of the preclinical phase, having attained the necessary entrance requirements. A small number of students pursue an intercalated year in order to pursue a preclinical science to honours degree standard before proceeding to their clinical studies. Students begin their clinical work in the fourth year of the course overall (which is thus the third actual year of study for the majority).

The fourth-year student's day begins with a lecture in a course on 'the nature of disease'. In the early weeks of the year, these lectures provide an 'introduction to clinical medicine', and include lectures on such general topics as: 'the approach to the patient': 'history-taking - the present complaint'; 'observation of the patient'. From then on the lecture course proceeds system by system, with talks from members of staff from various clinical and non clinical departments. This course of formal lectures on clinical topics is an attempt to provide a unifying element in an otherwise fragmentary clinical component.

After their lecture the students make their way to various clinical attachments in the teaching hospitals. The fourth year introductory teaching takes place in five of the hospitals associated with the university: the Royal Infirmary, the Western General, the Eastern General, the Northern General and the Leith Hospitals. During the first term of the year the fourth year students are all attached to medical units. In the second and third terms they are attached to a surgical unit and a second unit in medicine.

The groups in which the students are attached to medical and surgical units are known as 'cliniques', a term redolent of Edinburgh's close historical associations with the tradition of European medicine. In the first term, these groups (in medicine) contain about a dozen students. Later in the year the groups are rather smaller. These cliniques provide the students with a closely defined group of peers with whom they interact, with whom they work, and with whom they share their everyday experiences. Even though not all members of a clinique are close or even friendly before the group is formed at the start of a term, they become acquainted through sharing their clinical work. In these groups students negotiate their common views of shared problems, or debate their differences of opinion. On the wards, between teaching periods, in hospital canteens, waiting in corridors, on the coach between the university and an outlying hospital, the members of a clinique can chatter and reflect together on the teaching they are receiving, the patients they have seen, the characteristics of the clinicians and so on.

The general pattern of a clinical unit comprises male and female wards, a teaching room, the normal procedure rooms, doctors' and nurses' rooms and so on. Each clinical unit is staffed by a small number of consultants, plus their firm of registrars and housemen. The majority of such units are staffed by NHS clinicians, who hold honorary University appointments, or part-time teaching appointments. Some are University based units: the staff hold positions as professors, senior lecturers and lecturers, and have honorary appointments as consultants and registrars. These 'professorial' units tend to have larger complements of staff than their NHS counterparts.

One consultant described the arrangement of units as being 'like a series of cottage hospitals', referring to the degree of autonomy enjoyed by each. Each group of doctors takes the responsibility for arranging the teaching of the fourth year students, and for arranging this to fit in with their other work of patient care, research and administration. The particular staffing arrangements and practicalities of day-to-day organisation mean that the precise organisation and content of the teaching vary considerably from attachment to attachment. But there are common types of teaching that are generally found from unit to unit. These are the major types of clinical instruction and clinical encounter which are recognised and distinguished by staff and students themselves.

Bedside teaching. I have already presented a sketch of such teaching, and it is familiar. A doctor takes a group of students into the ward and teaches at a patient's bedside. The clinician may spend all of the time with just one patient, or conduct a 'round', teaching on a number of patients in succession. Such teaching provides occasion for students to learn and practise the techniques of history-taking and physical examination. Physicians and surgeons themselves can demonstrate such skills to the students. An individual patient and his or her problems may serve as a starting point for a more general discussion of pathology, clinical method, management and so on.

Tutorials. Doctors may conduct small group teaching sessions of a more theoretical nature, without direct recourse to the patients on the wards. These take place in the teaching rooms. On some units there are regular series of tutorials, on others they take place on an *ad hoc* basis. The teaching room may also be used for the discussion of points of interest that arise at the bedside and which the teaching clinician wishes to develop further; the room is often used as a backstage region in order to avoid discussing potentially worrying or distressing topics within earshot of the patient.

Waiting nights. The individual hospital units receive emergency admissions on a rota basis. On their receiving or waiting nights, fourth year students attached to a unit are expected to attend for at least part of the evening. Usually the students come in small numbers, members of the clinique taking it in turns to come in in twos and threes. On waiting nights the students are able to see patients who are admitted to the hospital in the acute phases of various conditions (such as myocardial infarctions in medicine, acute abdomens in surgery). Students have the chance to accompany doctors when they admit patients, see them take an initial history and examine the patient. They can be present when early differential diagnoses are formulated by the admitting doctor and management is initiated. On surgical attachments waiting nights provide opportunities for students to go into theatre, and observe operations taking place. The students may even have the chance to assist in the operating theatre, in a humble fashion, by holding a retractor.

Ward meetings. These occasions are not specifically designed as teaching occasions, but are, in a way, educational for all those concerned. Staff and students come together to discuss cases that they have on the wards. Cases are presented by senior students or members of staff, or someone may be asked to give a brief presentation on a specific topic of general interest. Rarely, a fourth year student may be asked to work up a patient for presentation. One of the pathologists may come to the meeting and discuss in detail the findings of biopsies, the results of post mortem examinations and so on. By and large the fourth year students take little active part in these meetings, though a doctor may pause to explain points of interest to them, ask them questions, check whether they understand the proceedings and so on.

Clerking. As well as seeing patients with clinical teachers in small groups, students may also be given the task of seeing patients individually. This activity, usually referred to as clerking a patient, is designed to allow students to take a full history and perform a full physical examination on a patient. When done thoroughly this takes the student a number of hours, possibly spread over a number of days, and on some days of the week a period of time is set aside (on some units) for students to get this work done on one or more patients. Members of a clinique may thus have patients allocated to them on a weekly basis - a list of students and 'their' patients is posted at the beginning of the week. On completion of the history and examination the students are usually required to write up the case notes and to formulate a differential diagnosis, as if they were responsible for the admission of the patient. The case notes are read and commented on by a staff member. From time to time a period may be set aside for the clinique members to go over the notes and findings together, and to present cases to each other.

The bedside teaching and clerking that are discussed here cannot be taken as typical of all British medical education in all its details. There has always been something of a difference in emphasis between the Scottish medical schools and their English counterparts (especially the London schools). In England the tendency has been to use the 'apprenticeship' system, with the student 'walking the wards', while in Scotland there has been an emphasis on small group teaching at the bedside. At Edinburgh students do not routinely become involved with the day-to-day care of individual patients. The form of clerking that they do is therefore an important way in which such involvement can be approximated on the wards. Since the students do not have responsibility for the care of patients, the main focus of the fourth year is a grounding for the students in basic clinical *method*. Emphasis is placed on students' acquisition of methods and routines of clinical inquiry. There is less emphasis placed upon management of patients and the practicalities of diagnostic or therapeutic work.

In addition to the general teaching arrangements already referred to, there is a range of other opportunities available to students. They may be able to attend post mortem examinations. At least one of the hospitals announced that such an event was taking place with a discrete notice *Sectio Hodie* (Autopsy Today). When students see the notice they are supposed to inform the clinician on their unit; if the dead person was one of their patients, and if it is thought 'interesting' or 'valuable', then the clinique attend the post mortem.

At times students attend outpatient clinics. They sit in on consultations between the doctor and the succession of patients whom he or she sees. The students may also be called upon to question or examine the patient themselves. There are, too, *clinical lectures* once a week in the Royal Infirmary for students in cliniques there. One of the consultants addresses the students in a lecture theatre. He may bring one or more of his own patients along from the wards in order to illustrate to them key features of the case. The patients who furnish the illustrative material for such lectures may be wheeled into the lecture theatre in their bed. Attendance at these lectures is rather patchy and many students 'skive off'. (They do feel constrained to attend the lecture if it is being delivered by a consultant from their own wards, lest their absence be noted and held against them.) Students often go along to these clinical lectures in order to 'have a look' at the various consultants, rather than seeing them as a major part of their clinical work. There is more than a hint of a theatrical display, in which the students learn more about the doctors' styles of performance than clinical medicine. In many ways these clinical lectures are the most ritualised among the ceremonial displays of clinical thaumaturgy. The consultant puts on something of a performance, using the patient's body as a key prop in that dramaturgical exercise.

One of the most dramatic and absorbing experiences for students in the fourth year is their early introduction to surgery. Although they do not necessarily take an active part in the actual performance of operations, the students get an opportunity to observe the work of the surgeons in the operating theatre. The theatres are equipped with galleries from which clinique members can watch what is going on. The surgeons can address remarks to the students, or provide a running commentary on the operation they are performing. Surgeons can stop and point out structures to the students, or quiz them on aspects of anatomy that they should know. Students may also observe from the floor of an operating theatre. It is, in fact, rather hard to see very much of what is going on during many operations. The small huddle of surgeons, anaesthetist and nurses blocks off a clear view of the action. The students often find themselves looking at the backs and bent heads of the operating team.

Rather like the first days in the anatomy dissecting rooms, a student's first operation may be seen as a major landmark in a student's growing repository of experiences. Like the introduction to anatomy, too, this experience is sometimes regarded with slight misgivings. But the novelty soon wears off, and it becomes one of the taken for granted things which students come to accept. These spectacles are also occasions for frustration, for the students' view is - literally - partial, and emphasises their marginal and subordinate status. Nonetheless, visits to the operating theatres do provide the students with valued opportunities for firsthand observations of the 'real' work of hospital surgery.

The precise arrangements for clinical work vary from unit to unit, but the general pattern is similar across them all. For students, the differences between cliniques are important, but the transition to clinical work is the most fundamental qualitative change that they recognise. While they have grumbles about aspects of their clinical work, the students are all agreed that it is preferable to the preclinical segment of the course. As one student expressed it:

> This year, the actual stuff isn't easier, but it's more interesting and it's easier to remember. When you see a patient with the disease process it's easier to remember; also it's easier to learn when you're taught in small groups.

Interest in the work of the clinical years is a recurrent theme in students' views of their time on the wards. One of the female students went so far as to say that she was now 'looking forward to Monday mornings', something that certainly had not been true during the earlier part of her course. For her things had been getting progressively better: the second year was 'shocking', the third year 'better', and as for the fourth year, she was actually 'enjoying it'. It was:

much more interesting than preclinical ... there's much less awful swotting. Because it's interesting I think you pick it up more easily.

For the students, this interest lies primarily in the perceived reality and relevance of their clinical studies, as opposed to the academic nature of the preclinical years. Dealing with patients is seen not only as inherently more interesting and absorbing, but also helping to put into perspective the material that has been (or should have been) assimilated in the second and third years. This is attributed to

The fact that you talk to patients, have actual contact with them, and the fact that you can see why you studied the stuff in the other three years makes it all worthwhile.

And as another student put it:

It's nice to have some contact with patients. You learn more by application this year than by rote, like we did last year.

Indeed, students would explain that sometimes they only really learned or understood some aspect of the preclinical syllabus when they began to encounter it in a clinical context. Anatomy and physiology particularly came into their own during the basic clinical training of the fourth year. In surgery, for instance, I often observed the surgeons 'revising' anatomy which they at least seemed to think the students should have known. Neuroanatomy and the anatomy of the peripheral vascular system, which were treated as important on at least some surgical units, were topics which students had to re-learn in the context of actual surgical problems and procedures.

It is not hard, of course, to see how the various scientific 'facts' could be learned more readily in the clinical context. Individual patients provide the most memorable of 'audio-visual aids' in the demonstration of illness. They furnish vivid exemplification, a dramatic enactment of medical concerns. On the basis of my own period of research, I can vouch for the memorability of clinical presentations. The individual patients I saw with the students remain fresh in my mind. For the students, their first patient with distinctive signs and symptoms of a particular disease remains fresh in the memory, in a way which the de-contextualised 'facts' of a textbook or the lecture theatre do not.

The fourth year students, then, welcome the move into the clinical phase as a shift towards the real work of medicine, and away from the academic, theoretical and scientific aspects of their course. Apart from periods of vacation work for some of them, the transfer marks the students' first sustained contact with practising doctors and their patients in the milieu of 'real' medical work.

The majority of students do not envisage entering non clinical medical work, such as research, epidemiology or public health. They see their eventual career involving direct contact with patients, either on hospital wards and clinics, or in general practice. While many do not have a precise specialty in mind, they are still committed to a future in clinical work of some sort. It is, therefore, hardly surprising that they should see the preclinical sciences as little better than something of a 'chore', a major hurdle to be negotiated before the 'real' work of medicine as such. The fourth-year students at Edinburgh certainly treat the division as a major one, and tend to look back on the preclinical years as drudgery. The overall course is long, and students are eager to complete it as rapidly as possible. The preparation for the 'Second MB' examination is looked back on by fourth years as a time of considerable emotional stress and intellectual effort. In comparison their introduction to clinical work seemed very easy and relaxed, apparently requiring much less sustained effort and concentration. As one of the female students put it, 'The third year was terrible; this year is much easier', and, as another said, 'You can go at a slower pace'.

The students' experience of work in the medical school is therefore paradoxical. They find themselves working heavily on matters which they do not find absorbing, or relevant to their future career; they feel less heavily committed when they come on to work which seems more central to their medical training. Ellis (1975) has remarked that in comparison with the 'tread-mill' of much of the undergraduate years, 'the long clinical course all too easily lacks any sense of urgency'.

The status passage from the preclinical years is welcomed by the students on two counts. Their new work is both easier, and more gripping. The organisation of the formal curriculum tends to imply that the preclinical years are to be thought of as preparation for more important work. The whole undergraduate curriculum appears to follow a simple logic: from the pure theory of the basic sciences to pure practical experience. The first clinical year therefore conveys the impression of a significant staging post in the sequence from theory to practice.

The clinicians themselves tend to reinforce this perception. They too stress a qualitative difference between the two phases. Rather than

23

continuity between the preclinical and clinical aspects, they tend to emphasise the fact that the students are 'starting again'. For instance, during the first week of my fieldwork one of the younger consultants on the medical unit I was observing told the clinique, 'You are in the delicate position of forgetting your physiology and learning medicine'. The following incident illustrates the general phenomenon:

> The students from various cliniques - about thirty of them - were taken for a demonstration of X-ray techniques. They all sat round and were invited to comment on a number of X-ray pictures that were put up at the front of the class, and to compare them with a 'normal' film which was also displayed. One girl made a suggestion that was, I gathered, way off target. Dr. Mason [one of the consultant physicians] commented to the radiologist, "They're allowed to say anything, you know; they don't know any medicine yet".

Just as the students find they need to re-learn their preclinical subjects in the context of bedside work, so the clinicians emphasise this to the students. In medicine, for instance, I noted that neurology was often described as little more than an applied knowledge of the underlying anatomy, and usually coupled with the criticism of the students' apparent ignorance of that anatomy. Similarly, the surgeons would often be at pains to rehearse basic anatomy while discussing operative techniques, discussing the findings of a particular case, looking at X-rays and so on.

As I shall go on to discuss in greater detail later, the clinicians would lay stress on clinical knowledge, contrasting it with both the theories of text books, and the teachings of non clinical scientists, to the detriment of the latter. For instance, a junior physician was teaching the students in a tutorial, and asked the students for the cause of a particular condition:

St: Myocarditis.
Dr: [derisively] Yah!
St: Well, that's the pathological description that's given for it.
Dr: Pathology's finished. We're on clinical work here; pathology's waffle, just cover-up stuff!

Similarly, I noted the following exchange between a consultant surgeon and the members of the clinique:

Dr: So there's an example of course of a goitre in a patient of thirty six - of long standing, eighteen years. So you are in a little difficulty if it isn't nodular. You've finished with thyroid pathology?

St: Yes

Dr: So what is it?

St: If it isn't nodular, it might be adenoma of the thyroid.

Dr: Hmm I sometimes think that pathologists have a distorted view of thyroid pathology. By adenoma I suppose you mean a simple tumour?

St: Yes.

Dr: Simple tumours of the thyroid are very rare.

The consultant then went to ask the students about the age of the onset of goitre:

St: Onset of puberty.

Dr: You're quite right that the text books talk of adolescent goitre, *but....*

and he went on to explain that the students should not rely on what the text books said on the matter.

In this particular exchange, the surgeon managed to contrast his own clinical approach both with the niceties of pathologists' theorising, and the received wisdom enshrined in text books. Such contrasts are by no means uncommon, and they provide a recurrent reinforcement of the primacy of clinical knowledge over 'theory'. Often such presentations of knowledge stress that the clinical is more down to earth, less concerned with pettifogging detail and exceptional cases. The clinician portrays himself as a pragmatist. Not, that is, that the clinician promotes a view of his knowledge as crude or unsophisticated; his is the subtlety of knowledge grounded in painstakingly accumulated personal experience.

In a number of ways, then, the students who enter their first clinical year feel that they have embarked on a novel and valuable segment of their careers. Many of them for the first time feel themselves gripped and absorbed by the world of real medicine that they now encounter. One young woman described her experience of the first term of clinical medicine as 'intoxicating', and many of her classmates too found it heady stuff.

This subjective experience of transition reflects what Davis (1968) has called the process of 'doctrinal conversion'. Davis seeks to capture 'those feeling states, inner turning points and experimental markings which, from the perspectives of the subject, impart a characteristic tone, meaning and quality to his status passage'. Davis draws on the very apt metaphor coined by Hughes (1958, p.119):

> One might say that the learning of the medical role consists
> of a separation, almost an alienation of the student from the
> lay medical world; a passing through the mirror so that one
> looks out at the world from behind it, and sees things as in
> mirror writing.

In all the more 'esoteric occupations', Hughes suggests, one finds this sense of seeing the world 'in reverse'. During the period of training and initiation, two cultures - the 'lay' and the 'professional' - interact. Hughes remarks that such interaction goes on throughout an individual's life:

> ... but it seems to be more lively - more exciting and
> uncomfortable, more self-conscious and yet perhaps more
> deeply unconscious - in the period of learning and
> initiation. (p.119)

In the professions, as Hughes observes, the process of 'passing through the mirror' is most apparent. The sense of difference, the sense of separation between the practitioner and the lay actor is most marked. Most studies of professional socialisation have tended to concentrate on how the novice comes to take on the appropriate perspectives and understandings, behaviour and values which characterise their newly-gained occupational culture.

Important though such concerns are, there has been a tendency to ignore or gloss over one crucial aspect of such occupational cultures, reflecting particular emphases on the processes of doctrinal conversion. While observers puzzle over the mysterious process whereby, say, medical students become doctors, they are in danger of overlooking one rather important component - that in the course of their years in medical school they learn medicine! Stated thus the observation seems quite absurdly trivial. But it is the case that what makes for the 'esoteric' nature of such occupations as medicine lies (in great measure) in the expertise which is their stock in trade. Irrespective of the actual, ultimate value of the occupation's accumulated wisdom, the knowledge and skills employed by practitioners form the cornerstone of their collective licence and mandate (cf. Hughes 1958). The acquisition of such competence underlies, too, the individual's subjective experience of doctrinal conversion. The medical student, after all, is not only taking on board values, attitudes and perspectives; he or she is engaged in the rapid - at times almost frenzied - accumulation of medical knowledge.

In the course of their training, students of the professions achieve some mastery over complex and powerful systems of explanation and understanding. They are powerful in the sense that they encompass many areas of personal and public concern, providing frameworks for interpretation and intervention in many aspects of everyday life. They are, of course, powerful too in the sense that they confer power, influence and prestige on those who manipulate them.

It is not surprising, therefore, that initiates should become fascinated by these realms of discourse and understanding. It has been noted in a number of different contexts that the vocabularies of expertise become incorporated into trainees' everyday accounts of themselves and others. Bucher and Stelling (1977, p.103), for instance, describe how one group of residents in psychiatry acquired and began to use their technical vocabulary to describe the supervisory process while talking about their relationships with superiors: 'There was an enormously detailed, elaborated description of each supervisor in terms of his character structure and the nature of his interaction and contribution to the supervision'.

In part, the use of such technical vocabularies in ordering experience can be seen as an element in 'role-playing' or 'role simulation'. Davis (1968), for instance, identifies simulation as a stage in the process of conversion, describing a 'genre of highly self-conscious, manipulative behaviour of students which aims at constructing institutionally valued performances of a particular role'. Students thus enact a somewhat uncertain version of what they take to be appropriate professional activity. This view, which is echoed by Olesen and Whittaker (1968) follows a fairly familiar dramaturgical view of the student actor, involved in 'psyching out' their teachers and presenting a front, or favourable self-presentation. Undoubtedly there is a good deal in this. Students do find themselves, more or less self-consciously, 'playing' at being doctors or nurses without feeling that they are really comfortable and at home in such activity. They subjectively experience themselves as occupying a 'liminal' position, neither fully competent experts nor still laymen. Yet to attribute students' use of their newly found, embryonic expertise simply to such manipulative role playing misses much of the students' experience.

In particular, the seductive appeal of much expert knowledge escapes such a perspective. As I have already indicated, it is part of the appeal of many bodies of esoteric knowledge that they furnish frames of reference which, apparently, account for many facets of human behaviour. They have connotations of revelation; they may offer insight into human motives, actions, problems and sufferings. The daily doings of one's fellows are a constant source of fascination, and the 'expert' is afforded privileged access to the private lives of others. Students gain firsthand experience of the troubles of a variety of people, while at the same time learning how to intervene in order to cure or alleviate them.

It is, therefore, small wonder that the novice, in the process of gaining competence in manipulating his or her developing expertise, should find them, quite literally, *absorbing*. Elsewhere, I have written, in a fairly lighthearted way, of the well-known phenomenon of 'medical students' disease' - that is, the hypochondria to which medical students are prone (Atkinson, 1977). It has been suggested that this is largely the outcome of heightened stress and anxiety on the students' part, in the face of extreme academic pressure. While this may play a part, I would prefer to suggest that all we need to postulate to account for students' hypochondria is not heightened anxiety, but a heightened awareness of the clinical. Students become more or less adept at handling a complex symbolic domain in which disease categories and diagnostic inference figure pre-eminently. It should therefore come as little surprise that clinical understanding should come to occupy a dominant position in students' repertoire of conceptual schemes. Certainly the fourth year students at Edinburgh applied candidate diagnoses to themselves as well as to others - to their teachers, at times, as well as to their patients. That they did so simply reflects the centrality of the clinical to the everyday experience of the student in her or his first clinical year.

It may be reasonable to account for such occasions as playful. Certainly students play with their stethoscopes, and with their tendon hammers. I often observed students engrossed in bashing their own knees with their hammers, producing repeated knee-jerks. But in describing it as play we should not assume that we are dealing with self-conscious, manipulative action: to do so overlooks the fact that in play we become absorbed, given over entirely to the activity in hand. The student who was 'intoxicated' with clinical work was describing something more totally gripping than simple simulation.

The fourth year students, in their initial encounters with clinical medicine, I am suggesting, become absorbed, seduced almost, by the clinical gaze. This particular doctrinal conversion occurs in the context of the teaching hospital, where the clinic is enacted, wherein the students are initiated into the mysteries of their craft. For students and staff alike, the importance of clinical, bedside teaching is self evident. Its legitimacy is guaranteed by virtue of the students' exposure to, and immersion in, the 'real world' of everyday life on the wards. In contrast with the abstract, academic worlds of the lecture theatre and the laboratory, on the hospital wards the students can engage directly with the very stuff of medicine. Its *authenticity* is thus self justifying. The rest of this book will be largely devoted to examining the nature of this clinical reality and its authenticity. My argument will be that this reality is artfully stage-managed. It is constructed so as to reproduce particular *versions* of medical work and a particular form of medical culture.

3 Researching the clinical milieu

Introduction

The initial impetus to study the Edinburgh medical school arose out of a mixture of biography and circumstance. I had originally gone to Edinburgh with the intention of working within a general framework of the phenomenology of language, an interest which derived from my reading of Alfred Schutz, an optional course in linguistics, and a course of lectures from Dell Hymes during my first degree in Social Anthropology at Cambridge. While casting about for a specific focus, I expressed an interest in the topic of typifications. It happened that Liam Hudson, my supervisor, had some unanalysed semantic differential data on medical students styereotypes of various occupational categories, including a number of medical specialties. Those semantic differential data had been collected some years previously at the London Hospital Medical School while the students were in their first year. It appeared that most of them would now be the final year students, and with the co-operation of John Ellis, then Dean of the London Hospital Medical School, comparable semantic differentials were distributed to the cohort.

I therefore spent some time analysing and writing up these semantic differential data. Interest in this approach was sustained at Edinburgh partly because of Hudson's own work on stereotypes of Arts and Sciences, and Coxon's work on the evaluation of occupational titles. In retrospect that particular methodology seems very crude and limited: I only ever published one *New Society* paper from those data, and much of the material remained unanalysed. It was, however, valuable experience in getting started on a research project, and it introduced me to medical students and their training. In the course of that initial inquiry, of course, I became familiar with the two classics of the sociology of medical education, *The Student Physician* (Merton *et al.*, 1957), and *Boys in White* (Becker *et al.*, 1961). Those whetted my appetite for a much more thorough investigation of medical education, not least because it appeared that no comparable research had been done in Britain. Ethnographic fieldwork was a particularly attractive proposition. Having initially been trained as a social anthropologist, I regarded fieldwork as the obvious way to set about research.

By the end of my first year as a research student, then, I had written a report on the London medical students' stereotypes, and had decided to try to embark on ethnographic fieldwork in the Edinburgh medical school. My general inspiration was a combination of a commitment to anthropological approaches to research, *Boys in White*, and the foreshadowed problem of medical students' typifications of different medical specialties.

In the event, the focus of the ethnography shifted: in common with many, if not most, ethnographers, I found that my foreshadowed problem became transformed, as I concentrated progressively on the conduct of clinical teaching in the students' first clinical years, in the specialties of Medicine and Surgery. My initial interest was not entirely lost to sight, however, since the students' reactions to Medicine and Surgery were intimately related to their typifications of physicians and surgeons.

Finding a way in

At the outset of my research it was quite clear that it would be impractical to try to cover the entire range of the Edinburgh Medical School: the resources and time at my disposal precluded such an approach. It was therefore necessary for me to scan the medical school, and to decide on some point of entry into the organisation and some vantage point from which to observe the students and their training. Several initial possibilities presented themselves. The first year of the curriculum was devoted primarily to basic sciences (Chemistry, Physics and Biology) and the medical content of the syllabus appeared to be limited. The second year seemed to afford greater possibilities: in this year the more distinctively 'medical' subjects were first encountered by the students - Anatomy, Biochemistry and Physiology. This period of the curriculum did appear to offer research possibilities, and I therefore spent some time, in a preliminary and rather haphazard way, joining the students in Anatomy and Physiology. Of particular interest at that time was my access to the Anatomy dissecting rooms, where I chatted to some of the students as they worked on their cadavers. The intrinsic and personal interest of this experience was considerable. Just as the experience of the dissecting room is often taken to be a necessary baptism for the new medical student: 'it is often taken for granted that getting used to dissecting is a major problem for freshmen, that first contact with dead bodies must be a difficult, if not traumatic, experience' (Becker *et al.*, 1961, p.102). As these authors note, it is a theme which frequently appears in fictionalised accounts of medical student life. Rosenberg (1969) described 'meeting the cadaver' as an occasion of stress among freshman medical students. The students I talked to in the dissecting rooms and on later occasions recounted their own misgivings and unease on first encountering their own cadaver - often with a sort of black humour - recounted at their own expense. There were one or two stories of students being unable to go through with dissection and withdrawing from the faculty. For most of them and for most of the time, however, the experience seemed to be assimilated in a matter-of-fact manner (cf. Becker *et al.*, 1961, p.103). Nevertheless I too took it as a personal initiation into the world of medicine. I had the half-articulated notion that if the medical students had to go through the symbolic *rite de passage* of the dissecting room then I too should share this most salient of their experiences. Although in the event this brief period in Anatomy did not form part of the research reported here, it did on occasion stand me in good stead with the students - in establishing my credentials with them.

In many ways, the brief period of fieldwork in Anatomy, and an equally short time in some Physiology classes, had a diffuse but significant intellectual effect. I have never explicitly drawn on data from those settings. Indeed, the Professor of Anatomy extracted from me the undertaking that I would not publish detailed accounts of the Dissecting Room: he suggested that future donors and their families might be dissuaded from bequeathing bodies for dissection if they read too vivid an account of the DR. I suspect he may have feared that an account might confirm some of the urban legends concerning the irreverent treatment of cadavers. It is no breach of my undertaking to indicate that I observed no such behaviour. Although I did not draw on my observations explicitly, and spent little time there, the experience of the Dissecting Room had an impact on me personally and on some of the analytic issues that I have returned to in subsequent years.

The Dissecting Room, with its rows of half-dismembered cadavers, is an extraordinary setting. It is far from repulsive or distressing, I found. (I have found the distress of the living much more unsettling than the mute, dismembered bodies of the dead.) In many ways, the contrary is the case: it has an intriguingly and unexpectedly uplifting effect. The generosity of those who had donated their bodies was inspiring. Moreover, the extraordinary intensity of the experience was moving. The human body is a fascinatingly complex organism. To be able to observe dissection at first hand provided a rare and privileged insight into the body and its structures. The experience also heightened one's awareness of the physical corporeality of the person, and - by extension - of one's self. The body, one appreciates, is not just a vehicle or medium for self-expression or self-presentation. The *physical* self and the body became central for my sociology of medical knowledge too. Having passed through Anatomy and Physiology with the students, I could not willingly reproduce the kind of sociology in which the patient is, paradoxically, disembodied. Equally, one could not study medical education and the reproduction of medical knowledge without paying due attention to how students and their teachers construe those bodies. The patient must be understood as a site of signs and symptoms, and the body is there to be investigated - observed, palpated, listened to, tapped, scraped, smelled and so on. In reporting on the reproduction of medical knowledge I have therefore tried to give due weight to the physical presence of patients' bodies and how medical students encounter those bodies.

Despite the interest and subsequent significance of those preliminary observations, I felt that I ought to focus my main research further on in the students' training. The students in Anatomy and Physiology were looking forward to their first contact with the work of clinical medicine, in the fourth year of the course. They saw the move from preclinical to clinical studies as a major landmark in their lives. The students' initial exposure to clinical work therefore suggested itself as a likely point for the examination of the development of students' views on the nature of medical work, and their perceptions of the various clinical specialties. My final decision, therefore, was to undertake a study of the fourth year - the first clinical year - by means of participant observation.

Getting started

Having decided that I wanted to concentrate on the first year of students' clinical studies and having committed myself to doing the research by means of participant observation and interviewing, I was then faced with the problem of negotiating access to the hospital wards. As it transpired, there was nothing inherently difficult in this, but it was a protracted process. My negotiations really began with Professor Archie Duncan, the Professor of Medical Education and Executive Dean of the Medical Faculty. Had it not been for his interest and support of my research - at least in the form it took - would not have got off the ground. It was he who sponsored my application for permission to spend time with the students on the hospital wards. There was some problem insofar as the methodology of participant observation was rather alien to the scientific outlook of the members of the Medical School staff. Research on medical students and their education is by no means unusual, and much of the British research had been done in Edinburgh. But the research paradigms employed tended to rely heavily on the administration of attitude surveys, or personality inventories. The emphasis was very strongly on the quantitative approach to such research. My approach did not square with the normal expectations of worthwhile research, and seemed 'woolly' and 'subjective'.

In the event a formula was found which satisfied the sensibilities of the Faculty members. The minutes of the Faculty meeting which approved my research proposal gave me permission to associate unobtrusively with groups of students, on the understanding that this would in some sense be a preiiminary strategy until I formulated more detailed proposals. In the event, once this general approval had been granted, it became apparent that such further details were not required, until at the end of the first year of the project I distributed a questionnaire to the students. The draft questionnaire was submitted in advance to the Executive Dean. This was the extent of the further involvement of the Medical Faculty in the conduct of the research. It was made a condition of my fieldwork that I could mingle with the larger clinique groups, and that therefore association with students in their final year, who are attached to clinical units individually or in small numbers, was ruled out. Obviously such a condition did nothing to hamper my work with the fourth-year students.

The permission granted by the Faculty also made it clear that my actual participation in medical work was dependent upon the permission of the relevant Head of Department, and of the doctors on the individual clinical units. Thus even though the initial hurdle had been cleared, I was still faced with a number of further negotiations before I could actually join the students on the wards. The Faculty of Medicine office sent out a duplicated letter from the Executive Dean, introducing me and reproducing the Faculty minute that gave me permission to go ahead. For my second year's work, in surgery, this letter was suitably modified and sent to the staff members of the surgical units.

For my first unit in medicine, I had already made contact with some of the staff members, via introductions from another member of the medical school staff. Thereafter, in order to gain access to further units I simply asked the senior consultant of each firm for his permission to join his students. Although I was from time to time warned that individual consultants might prove difficult and be unwilling to let me come and spend time in their wards, I was in fact refused access by only one of the consultants I approached. Since there were far more clinical units than I could cover anyway, seventeen in all, this one refusal did not in any way hamper or hold up the research as a whole. The beginning of the research was not without its crises, however. I learned that a number of consultants were somewhat concerned about my presence in the teaching hospitals, and there was talk of bringing the matter before the Board of one of the Hospitals. The General Medical Council was also mentioned darkly. Luckily, however, senior members of the staff were able to allay their most pressing misgivings.

For the most part, the chiefs of the various firms did not lay down any strong conditions on my research, and none of them subjected me to the sort of searching 'grilling' that I had rather expected. In making my requests for access I found it remarkably difficult to explain to the doctors what it was that I was planning to do on their wards. However, I found that they themselves readily translated my stumbling outline into the general formulation of 'communication' - between doctors and students, and between students and patients. I believed that this formulation of theirs adequately covered what I wanted to observe, and that in agreeing to it as a description of my research interests I was not guilty of any serious misrepresentation. This interpretation of my research project was also voiced as I did the research. For instance, during my work in medicine I noted:

> Dr. McDonald then came into the teaching room. Before he began to teach he turned to me, and explained that the students would shortly be looking at case-history notes, and as yet did not know about the normal ranges and values for haematological reports. He was therefore going to take a tutorial on the interpretation of haematology lab. reports. He went on to say to me that there would be 'no fancy patient-contact stuff - it's all meaty stuff'.

It was also a recurrent perception on the part of clinicians that I was involved in some explicitly evaluative exercise. It was a common reaction to take it that I was involved in action-research which was directly and immediately oriented to the formulation of improved teaching practices on the clinicians' part. For example, one senior registrar in medicine confided in me that he welcomed my presence and the research I was doing. He had, he explained, been in the army and he was worried, as he felt that he could teach the assembly and maintenance of a bren-gun much better than he could teach on a patient. He was worried over his own teaching, and the nature of clinical instruction in general. I tried to disabuse him of the notion that I was sufficiently expert in educational theory and methods to offer any immediate advice in this area. But other doctors would occasionally defer to me as an 'educational expert' - for instance when propounding some pet educational theory of their own to the students they would stop and seek my approval for their ideas. On such occasions I was forced to equivocate; in the context of a teaching occasion I was not able to go into any lengthy discussions of my research, its methods and its implications.

Students would likewise formulate their own interpretations of what my research might be about. The most usual solution also lay in the assumption that mine was an evaluative research project. They took it that I was evaluating clinical teaching in general, the approach of individual teachers, or both. They therefore expected me to be able to make comments on the 'efficiency' of bedside teaching as an educational method, or the nature of small-group dynamics at the bedside and in the tutorial room. Although I would try to explain that I was not directly involved in evaluation, I was never able to convince some of the students fully that this was the case. They tended to assume that I was interested in their experiences on their clinical attachments (as indeed I was) as evidence of those units' educational merit: the information that students volunteered on this score served the purpose of my developing research concerns, however, despite being based on false premises.

Day-to-day negotiations

Although I found that it was relatively straightforward to be granted permission to attend clinical teaching periods, this did not mean that my day-to-day presence on the wards was unproblematic. Quite apart from the senior consultants concerned, I also had to negotiate with the various teachers who were engaged in the bedside instruction. This was not straightforward. In the first place, I found that although chiefs of firms would assure me that they would inform their colleagues of my imminent arrival on their wards, this was not always done, and I would find that after my first interview with the chief, I might go out of his head almost immediately. Even when the doctors had been forewarned, the news did not always filter through to all members of the staff - and the more junior doctors might well have been left uninformed. Consequently, I would find that I was going in 'cold' with little or no prior warning for the doctors concerned. Very often the arrangements for my introduction had to be *ad hoc*, when I arrived on the wards. On my first morning on one of my medical attachments, I noted:

When I first went onto the wards I was not at all sure what sort of reception had been laid on for me, although I had already negotiated general access with the chief of the service. When I arrived, I found that the students were about to spend the first hour of the morning in individual ward work. As I was not entirely sure of my welcome, I stopped a passing doctor (whom I did not recognise) and asked him who was in charge of the students' work that morning. He told me to go and see Dr. Foster, who was upstairs. I went upstairs to the other ward; I found the ward sister and asked for the Doctor. She went away, came back and asked me to wait. I had to wait quite some time.

It appeared that Dr. Foster himself was busy with his clinical work, and as I waited in the corridor I could see him bustling in and out of one of the small single rooms just inside the ward doors.

After some ten or fifteen minutes, Dr. Foster came out to speak to me .... He seemed quite affable, and told me that I could join the students for their ward work now if I wanted to. In fact I decided that it would be tactless to butt in in the middle of the students' history-taking. (I had had to wait until after 10.30 to see Dr. Foster.) So I hung about in the doctor's room.

In the room I was quickly confronted with the necessity of entering into a new introduction and negotiation. After I had been there some minutes, one of the consultants came in with two housemen. Whilst I hovered in the corner, Dr. Robinson (I could read his name from his label badge) and his junior staff entered into a discussion at the other end of the room. Dr. Robinson was going through a pile of case-notes and he appeared to be discussing patients with a view to teaching on them. I could not hear all that was being said, but I could hear Dr. Robinson talking about patients as suitable 'teaching material', and at one point seemed to be discounting one patient for teaching purposes, as the clinical findings were 'not clear enough'.

When Dr. Robinson had finished, he turned, looked shrewdly in my direction and confronted me. 'Do I recognise you?' he asked. I told him my name and indicated briefly why I was there. I gathered from his reception of me that he had heard of me, and he seemed quite satisfied. He seemed at this first meeting to be a very pleasant and agreeable doctor.

On this occasion I was able to start observing and to start my ongoing negotiations more or less at the same time. Although I had made detailed arrangements of when I was going to start work on the unit with the chief, even the consultant I first met appeared to have only the most vague impression that I was expected on the wards. I had a similar sort of reception on my first surgical attachment. The very first session on my first Monday morning had been taught by the chief of the firm himself. But, as I recorded subsequently, his memory for my identity was remarkably short.

When the students all went off for coffee at about 11.15 I stayed behind, hoping to find whoever was going to teach the next session and introduce myself to him. I therefore hung about, and stopped the chief as he emerged from the doctors' room. I asked if he knew who was taking the next session, so that I could introduce myself. 'Yes', he replied, 'Who are you?'

'Paul Atkinson'

'Of course'. He put his arm round my shoulders and led me into the doctors' room, where a number of the surgeons were having their morning coffee. He introduced me very briefly, 'This is Mr. Atkinson, who is doing a survey of surgical teaching.' Then he left me ....

I asked one of the consultants if he knew who would be teaching the next period with the fourth year students, and he told me that it would be a Mr. Jenkins. I misinterpreted a non-verbal cue from the consultant and thought that one of the other surgeons present was the said Mr. Jenkins. Discovering my mistake (and feeling even less at ease) I then asked if Mr. Jenkins was around. Mr. MacKay said he was 'down in S.C.D.' and that they themselves would be going there shortly. When he had finished his coffee, he took me downstairs, to what turned out to be the Surgical Consultation Department (i.e. an out-patient department). He went into one of the little consultation rooms and brought out Mr. Jenkins, whom he introduced to me, and who readily agreed to my joining his teaching session.

Unobtrusiveness and social relations in the field

Although my presence on the wards had originally taken a fair amount of negotiation, once access had been agreed, I was generally taken very much for granted by the doctors on the wards, and by the students as they went about the hospital. Essentially, I was left to get on with what I wanted. Indeed, for some doctors I became so much a part of the normal scene that they forgot who I was: on several occasions I was taken for a student. For example:

> We went to the ward, to find Dr. Morrison waiting by the entrance to the ward. He told us to hurry up, and there was a sort of benign asperity and gruffness about his voice. There were still some of the clinique members away at coffee, and we stood about waiting for them. Somebody again mentioned the graduation ceremony that had just taken place, and the degree of B.Sc.Med.Sci.. Dr. Morrison then asked the students I was with if any of them had taken the degree. They were mostly second-year entrants and so had not done so. Dr. Morrison then turned to me and said 'Are you a B.Sc. Medical Sciences?'
>
> 'No, B.A. Cantab', I replied.
>
> 'Oh, we should call you "sir"! What made you choose Edinburgh as your medical school?'
>
> I briefly reminded Dr. Morrison of who I was - pointing out that I had already been to see him to explain about my research and to introduce myself. I told him that I had assumed that he had recognised me again, and that I wasn't trying to fool him in any way, or to join the group furtively. Dr. Morrison then appeared to remember who I was, and took no further notice of me.

39

This interaction with Dr. Morrison was not the only one in which my presence with the students - which I thought had been registered and taken as read by the doctor - was suddenly questioned in this way. One such incident occurred with a physician whom I had already met on more than one occasion. He was teaching the students round the bed of a very old lady, who was unconscious. The patient was in one of the small single rooms which opened off the entrance to the main open ward. As there was not a lot of room in there, I tried to keep out of the way of the students. There was in any case little to see, and there seemed no point in my crowding in. The patient was lying on her side, with her face turned towards the wall. At one point in the proceedings the clinician wanted the students to get really close to the head of the bed and observe the patient's eyes. As they all crowded into that corner, I hung back at the foot of the bed - as I thought, being considerate. After a moment or two the physician noticed me there, broke off what he was saying to the students and said to me 'You won't see very much from down there'. Although his tone was rather sharp, I still assumed that he realised who I was. I replied 'Oh, it's all right, thanks, I can see all I need to ....'. The doctor then made it clear that he had misunderstood the situation, and had taken me for a student, and that my reply sounded very inappropriate. I hastily reminded him that I was there to observe the bedside teaching, and of who I was. 'Oh!' he said, 'You're not tape-recording all this, are you?' When I told him that I was not, he seemed perfectly happy, and paid no further attention to me throughout the rest of the teaching session.

Although it was a regular part of my negotiations for access that patients should be made aware of my presence and the reason for my being there, such information was in fact never vouchsafed to the patients. But from time to time I became aware that the patients were noting my presence, and were looking at me rather quizzically: I neither taught, nor did I answer any questions. Sometimes I felt that I must have stuck out from the rest of the group. However, there was only one occasion when my presence was openly queried by a patient. It happened on a medical unit, when my fieldwork was quite well advanced, in the third term of the first year. I was with one of the consultants and three of the students. The group were all seated round a patient's bed, and I sat behind the students, towards the foot of the bed. I was visible to the patient, but not in direct line of vision as she spoke to the rest of the clinique. My position was, I felt, sufficiently unobtrusive, and I took some notes as the students took turns in questioning the patient. The patient herself was a middle-aged woman, bright yellow with jaundice. As the students' questioning progressed, it became apparent that the woman drank heavily - and indeed that she was probably an alcoholic. Throughout the teaching session the woman's attitude towards the consultant, and to the whole exercise, was one of detached boredom - of *belle indifference*. She appeared to lack any interest in her own condition. At the same time, she did appear to feel free to pass comment on the proceedings, and to take the initiative in starting new lines of conversation (often quite alarmingly tangential to the doctor's and students' lines of inquiry). For instance, at one point:

> The patient interrupted again saying, 'One thing is different. I know I'm not asking the questions, but last time I had my own cutlery and crockery - which I haven't had this time - which my doctor said I should have - as it might be - what's the word?...'

Later, the consultant and the students moved on to a discussion of possible causes and signs of obstructive jaundice. Whilst they were talking amongst themselves, the patient broke in:

> 'What about the little man at the back - I can't see his face!' I shifted slightly so that she could see me a bit, and gave her a little smile. Dr. Maxwell laughed and told her 'He's our scribe - he's writing it all down'. The patient herself seemed to have lost interest again.
>
> Dr. Maxwell and the students discussed possible clinical signs among themselves. The patient seemed quite uninterested, and was whistling quietly to herself.
>
> I took care to let her see me from time to time, making sure I did not catch her eye too much, and so spark off new tangents in her comments.

This particular patient was rather unusual. At one point Dr. Maxwell interrupted the history-taking and took the students aside to comment on how odd she was being. Her indifference and ironic detachment marked her off from the normal run of the patients I saw. When the teaching session was over, the consultant commented to me 'She was an odd bird. She picked you up!' Of course, it is noticeable that even this patient, who asked directly who I was, hardly received a full explanation for my presence.

Unobtrusiveness could prove rather difficult. At times I could be taken for a student, and 'put on the spot' by a doctor who mistook me for one. This became particularly noticeable in surgery, when I went into the theatre with the students. If we were in an open theatre, rather than behind a glass screen, we all had to put on gowns, caps and masks. With only our eyes showing it became difficult to recognise who was who - only a student's gender was apparent (and that was not always totally obvious under the voluminous theatre gowns). Under such conditions I became especially vulnerable to problems of 'mistaken identity' - I was acutely aware that I might be picked on suddenly to answer a question thrown out by the surgeon at the table. For instance, shortly after observing an operation to remove part of a patient's thyroid, I wrote:

> When he had removed the second part of the goitre, Mr. MacDonald said to the gallery, 'Perhaps one of you would like to go up to the frozen section with it ....' as he handed the bowl with it in to the theatre porter. Mr. MacDonald looked up, and suggested that one of the two students on the end of the rows would be easiest. Since I was sitting at the end of the row, I was one of the two. I was by no means sure that in looking up Mr. MacDonald knew who I was, and I was very unwilling to go through any further negotiation and explanations - either with the pathologists, or in the presence of the theatre staff. I therefore nodded to the other student and indicated with my head that he should be the one to go out, whilst the group of students looked round at each other, in some indecision. Luckily the other student went off to take the specimen away. I am not sure whether *he* recognised me either. This is obviously one of the perils of wearing surgical masks!

Field roles

It has often been customary to describe the performance of ethnographic research in terms of a role that is adopted by the researcher in the field (cf. Schatzman and Strauss, 1973). However, it is not possible to designate my position in the field in terms of any single, stable role. This can be illustrated by reviewing briefly the ideal-typical role descriptions that have been devised by methodologists in an attempt to capture the degree of participation and involvement with the action in the settings observed. A classic exposition of this was that of Gold (1958), who identifies four such roles: 'complete participant'; 'participant-as-observer'; 'observer-as-participant'; 'complete observer'. The so-called 'complete participant' is typified as operating under conditions of role pretence: his or her true identity and the purpose of the research are not disclosed. An example of this research strategy is that adopted by Lofland and Lejeune (1960) in their study of Alcoholics Anonymous. Complete participation may also characterise research based on unpremeditated participation or enforced presence in certain situations, where research is not the reason for the sociologist's presence; examples of the retrospective reporting of such participation are Davis's period as a cab-driver (Davis, 1959), or Roth's enforced period of observation in a tuberculosis sanatorium (Roth, 1963). The deliberate deceptions which are an inescapable aspect of the first of these approaches raise serious ethical problems, and some of these will be taken up in my later discussion of the ethics of my own research.

The complete observer role is rarely encountered in ethnographic research - at least in a pure form or as a dominant technique in any given research enterprise. In adopting this strategy the fieldworker is entirely removed from interaction with those he or she observes. Such an approach can be used most easily and efficiently for the observation of behaviour in public places, in relatively anonymous social settings. Insofar as it is not anchored in a detailed knowledge of the settings and the participants, it can be used to cover a wide range of situations. However, for any research in more private domains, where access is not automatically granted to all and sundry, it is not normally available to the researcher. The exigencies of negotiating access and sustaining relations in the field will normally necessitate that the researcher adopt a less detached role in the field. As Schatzman and Strauss (1973) commented:

> ... observing without being observed is virtually impossible
> to manage in natural social settings. The need to sit in on
> relatively private discussions, and to ask questions,
> precludes this tactic as a reasonable option. (p.59)

Schatzman and Strauss (1973) also emphasized the extent to which 'unobtrusive deportment' is something that must be worked at by the researcher, and made situationally appropriate:

> The researcher may sit in the corner of a room and not
> enter into conversation. The flow of events is not
> appreciably influenced by his activity .... But this option
> poses some dangers: the spectre of a relatively impassive

observer whether or not taking notes, barely showing appropriate affect or active curiosity, and offering few if any cues as to what he is 'really up to', can be very disturbing to the hosts. This option cannot be carried on indefinitely and universally for all situations. (p.59)

'Complete' observation, with no interaction, is therefore practically inefficient in many settings. In others it is a fallacy to believe that it is even possible. In the context of my own research, complete observation vis-à-vis all the participants on the hospital wards was a total impossibility. However, as I have just discussed, the degree of participation which marked my research varied from one category of observed actors to another, and from one social setting to another.

The varieties of observer-as-participant and participant-as-observer are more frequently approximated in the performance of field research. In both cases, the observed are aware of the nature of the researcher's identity and purpose. The distinction that Gold draws between the two varieties depends upon the emphasis placed on close interaction and participation with the research hosts. The observer-as-participant remains a relative stranger to the group members, and is something of an outsider: the participant-as-observer becomes more closely involved in the conduct of their daily lives and their interactions.

Both of the extreme or pure types of field strategy described have their drawbacks - and they are very similar. In neither case does the researcher have much leeway in managing interpersonal relations. The ability to question actors about their activities may be curtailed in both contexts, and approaches based on interviewing will often be ruled out, lest one's inquisitiveness lead to suspicion, or one's cover is blown. The complete participant may find physical and social access in the field setting limited by the nature of the assumed role. For instance, if, in the conduct of medical research, the ethnographer should adopt the role of a hospital porter, or similar auxiliary worker, then the ability to move and converse freely will be limited by the customary rights and duties attendant upon that chosen role. The complete observer by definition is denied possibilities: access to backstage areas, inner sanctums and so on, will normally be denied without disclosure of his or her identity and interests. The intermediate types of strategy normally allow the researcher to be a great deal more flexible; one will normally be able to range over a variety of situations, and be more free to investigate events by questioning in the field, or by means of interviews afterwards.

While such role definitions provide a handy way of conceptualising social relationships in the field, they have never captured the range of negotiations and roles that the researcher may have to perform. Descriptions like those of Gold tend to present a picture of an undifferentiated social milieu. Yet in complex organisations such as a hospital or medical school, this is not so. There are many categories of members - differentiated by their occupational specialisation, their place of work or sphere of influence, and their grade within occupational hierarchies. It is not necessarily the case that research will be directed towards all these organisation members equally. In my own case, I was primarily orientated towards the medical students, and my contacts with other medical school and hospital personnel were contingent upon that main focus. Consequently the extent to which I was a disengaged observer or a participant in the action depended on the nature of the particular group I was with, and the nature of the occasion. I was always an observer of the nursing staff and auxiliary personnel: I was a much more involved participant with some groups of students, whilst with others I remained a much more marginal figure.

The give-and-take of negotiations in the field mean that it may be expedient - and may come quite naturally - for the observer to become an engaged participant for brief periods. As a researcher it is always easy to find oneself rather aloof from others, always *taking* from one's informants and never giving. A lack of reciprocity can create strain and difficulty in one's field relations and these feelings may be rectified by the occasional participation in activities. Such occasional participation has been described as 'the-engaged-observer-as-transitory-participant'. Participation of this sort arises when the researcher can help out in various ways. For instance, during my early days in the field I was with a class of students who were first learning to use an ophthalmoscope. They paired off and took it in turns to look into each other's eyes with the instrument. There was an odd number of students in the group, and one of them ended up with no partner. It was therefore a natural action for me to offer to stand in and let him examine my eyes. In the same way in surgery I offered to act as a lay figure for a teaching session; I volunteered to play the part of the patient while students learned to drape me in preparation for an operation. Such participation helps to sustain the give and take of rapport in the field.

Students would sometimes make bids to engage me in more active giving which were more problematic. By virtue of my research topic, they would try to involve me as an expert on aspects of the medical school. They would try to use me as a source of inside information about the nature and the quality of the teaching offered in different teaching hospitals, or by different doctors. As I discuss later, such information is an important resource among the student body and is a recurrent topic of conversation: I offered an additional source for such evaluations. Such bids for involvement were less easy to acquiesce to, since I was usually concerned to discover the students' opinions or expectations of other clinical units and clinicians, rather than peddling my own opinions. Additionally, of course, there was the problem that such disclosures could get back to faculty members, and create an unfavourable impression. It was usually possible to deflect students' bids for information. I could plead my research interest in refusing to gossip about teachers and teaching - pointing out that it might constitute a breach of confidentiality and threaten the smooth progress of the research. I would also point out that what *I* thought was far less interesting than what *they* thought. When I did pass on tit-bits of information to students or groups of students, it was always with the specific aim of testing their reactions to it.

Watching, listening and recording

My periods of field observation were normally the hours of clinical work from ten o'clock to one o'clock each day. I spent those three hours accompanying the students on whatever activities were scheduled for them. This allocation of time was an extremely satisfactory one. The morning period was usually an active one, and required lengthy periods of concentrated observation: the afternoon was then free to write up the notes and observations of the morning. This is an important consideration. The span of memory for field observation is short and it is important that the notes should be written as soon after the event as possible, and certainly within twenty-four hours (Lofland, 1971). By confining the observation to the morning's teaching I was thus able to make this aspect of the research manageable.

During the time I spent in the hospitals I had no hard and fast methods of data collection. I found that my strategies for observation and recording changed as the nature of the social scene changed. Whenever possible I attempted to make rough notes and jottings while I was in the field. Such notes were then amplified and added to later in the day when I returned to the office. The quantity and type of on-the-spot recording varied across recurrent types of situation. During tutorials, when one of the doctors taught the group in a more or less formal manner, or when there was some group discussion, and conducted in one of the teaching rooms, then it seemed entirely natural and appropriate that I should sit among the students with my notebook on my knee and take notes almost continuously. At the other extreme, I clearly did not sit with my notebook and pen whilst I was engaged in casual conversation with students over a cup of coffee. Whereas taking notes during a University class is a normal thing to do, taking notes during a coffee-break chat is not a normal thing. To have done so openly in the latter context would have been to strain the day-to-day relationships that I had negotiated with the students. Whilst I never pretended that everything I saw and heard was not data, it would not have been feasible to make continuous notes. As Lofland has pointed out, the practice of participant observation must always involve a degree of betrayal:

> It happens that participants everywhere do and say many
> things they would prefer to forget or prefer not to have
> known, or at least not widely known. In the process of
> writing up his notes, the observer necessarily violates these
> participant preferences.   (Lofland, 1971, p. 108)

Such betrayal is probably an inescapable part of doing research of this sort, and the collection of such off the cuff remarks and observations meant that the notebook normally remained in the pocket, to be resorted to only afterwards.

Less clear-cut was my approach to the observation and recording of bedside teaching. On the whole I tried to position myself at the back of the student group and make occasional jottings: main items of information on the patients, key technical terms, and brief notes indicating the shape of the session, (e.g. the sequence of topics covered, the students who were called on to perform and so on). As I did this over a period I discovered that a substantial amount of the interaction could be recalled and summarised from such brief and scrappy jottings. Schatzman and Strauss make the same point in their discussion of field work technique:

> A single word, even one merely descriptive of the dress of
> a person, or a particular word uttered by someone usually
> is enough to 'trip off' a string of images that afford
> substantial reconstruction of the observed scene.
> (Schatzman and Strauss, 1973, p. 95)

During the first days of the research I found that I was producing 'filled in' field notes of a very general kind, describing broad features of the action-scenes I had observed. As the research progressed, I found I was able to observe more selectively, and hence take more detailed notes on brief episodes of the interaction. I was then able to spend the time in noting the direct speech on the spot and using the reconstruction after the event to provide contexts for these sequences of talk.

There is a constant problem that faces the fieldworker: what should be sacrificed. A complete description would be well-nigh endless, and a degree of selectivity must be employed. During the first days in the field, one is, willy-nilly, selective in reporting. A great deal that happens appears at first sight to be of little consequence, and its significance is easily lost on the naive observer. The initial problem is thus finding and remembering something worth saying. Later I began to focus on a number of key issues. The problem of selectivity was to some extent resolved through the development and emergence of substantive themes in the collection and organisation of the field data.

There were some mornings when I sacrificed observation for recording. It sometimes happened that events which occurred during the first half of the morning and afterwards during the coffee break would seem too good to miss. If I found that I had a great deal of action and talk that I wanted to record as quickly as possible, and in as much detail as I could, then I would sometimes stay on in the hospital canteen, and over additional cups of coffee, spend further time in writing field notes and reflecting on what had been said and done. The balance between the quantity of observation and the quality and depth of the subsequent writing is always an important and tricky element in the development of a field strategy. In the case of my own fieldwork I would sacrifice further observation if I felt that in monitoring the morning's activities, I had made some sort of breakthrough. It might be that something had happened that illuminated a series of earlier events, or aptly illustrated some point that I was striving to understand. Such occasion thus seemed to require more immediate and detailed recording than might be the case if I postponed writing up the notes, and confused the issue with yet more observation. I worked on the assumption that a bird in the hand was worth two in the bush, in that one well recorded event was worth more than two half-remembered and less well reported periods of observation.

The extent of the observations

During the first year of the research, I spent the best part of all three terms of the academic year in the field. I attended two medical units during the first term, a further two during the second term, and one more in the third term. The following year I spent the second and third terms observing surgical work. Over the spring term I attached myself to two surgical units, and in the summer term I attended an additional surgical unit. (There was no fourth-year teaching of surgery in the autumn term.)

I did not spend every available day observing on the wards: in general I tried to spend between three and four weeks with each unit. I did attempt to put in an appearance on the wards on every day of that period, even if I was not with the students all morning. The allocation of time was a reflection of my attempt to achieve some degree of balance between breadth and depth of coverage. As my field work got under way, it became apparent that the distinctive styles of the individual clinical units, and the contrasts between them was an emergent and dominating theme in students' discussions and their preoccupations. I was therefore eager to sample a range of different units for myself. At the same time, it was clear that there was insufficient time to attach myself to all the available clinical firms. A period of at least a few weeks were needed to cover the activities of a firm. In some cases, there were consultants who taught only one period a week, or there were student activities that were scheduled for only one day a week. To achieve even a limited acquaintance with these aspects of the work of a clinical unit, a stay of several weeks was necessary. However, I also found that by the end of a month of daily participation and observation, many of the features of life in the unit which had appeared distinctive were tending to become familiar, and that the freshness of my perceptions of the unit was starting to wear off. When such a sense of the familiar became apparent, I would try to move on to a new unit. By such moves I was forced to make the necessary changes in perception and understanding which threw the most routine affairs into a new relief.

Obviously, the timing of my fieldwork was determined by the calendar of the academic year. There was no necessity for me to decide just when to enter the field and when to leave it. Whereas some writers on participant observation have noted the problem of 'closure' - of when it is time to leave the field and terminate the observations - I was presented with something of a *fait accompli*. At the end of each term, and finally at the end of the academic year, there was no problem of how to stop my work with the students - they all disappeared anyway. In the same way, the beginning of each new term provided me with ready-made points of entry into a new clinical unit. Since it was the students' first day in the new milieu, it was easier for me to establish myself as part of the scene. For the units that I joined at the beginning of a new term, there were fewer problems in becoming accepted and establishing my presence, than with those groups I had to join midway through a term, when they had already had time to establish themselves in the attachment.

By concentrating on just one year of the undergraduate medical course - a critical year, as I saw it - I was able to achieve a degree of detail and intensity of analysis that was, I believe, reflected in the resulting ethnography. Had I attempted a diachronic analysis of socialisation in the medical school, I should have had to deny myself access to the fine grain of everyday life in any of the years or locales in the medical school. Whilst larger research teams, like that of Becker and his colleagues (Becker *et al.*, 1961), can realistically attempt more grandiose schemes of that sort, a single year's course is more suited to the one-man-band type of operation. From this point of view it is instructive to compare Miller's study of a small group of interns (Miller, 1970) with the study of Kansas medical school. Miller's study was explicitly designed to be a parallel to the latter monograph, and in many ways resembles a scaled-down version of *Boys in White*. The difference in the degree of coverage, in the bulk of data, and in sheer 'weight' reflects the different resources available for the two projects.

My allocation of time provided for a naturalistic sampling. My contact was mainly with the groups of students attached to the various cliniques, whose day-to-day experiences I was observing. Thus I was able to relate their talk (e.g. during interviews) to the social and educational context in which their experiences had been located. It was within these clinique groups that the students' perspectives on the nature of their clinical work were debated and negotiated.

Ethics, medical and sociological

Both the method and the subject matter of the research raise questions of ethics. My presence on the wards, insofar as I was not medically qualified or a medical student myself, was something which raised problems of professional ethics in my dealings with a number of clinicians. As I have already outlined, during the initial phases of my access negotiations, I was informed that a few of the senior consultants had heard of my projected research and were voicing reservations. These were couched in terms of doubt as to whether my presence could be justified, or even permissible, in terms of the ethics of medical practice. During the preliminary negotiations with the Department of Medicine, such misgivings were eventually allayed, and none of the physicians I approached withheld their general permission to join their cliniques. However, during my later negotiations with the surgeons, although general permission had been forthcoming from the Department of Clinical Surgery, one consultant did explicitly deny me access to his wards on the basis of medical ethics. It was, he told me, contrary to his interpretation of his professional code of conduct to allow me to attend his ward rounds: he added that he found it hard to understand why the medical school should have agreed in principle to my research proposals.

More generally, the problem of medical ethics cropped up only sporadically. One consultant on a medical unit took me aside and explained to me on the first morning that I met him that he was unhappy about my presence with the students: his Hippocratic oath, he explained, permitted him to demonstrate only to those who were 'apprenticed to the art'. He added that his reservations were reinforced that morning by virtue of the fact that he intended teaching on a female patient. On that occasion I explained to him that I had no intention of placing him in a difficult position and volunteered to withdraw from the morning's teaching round. I did so with as good a grace as I could manage. It appeared that the problem of exposing a female patient before a layman was of more importance than the general ethical position, as I was subsequently permitted to accompany the same consultant on teaching rounds.

This problem of female patients provided me with some uneasiness on my very first morning on one medical unit. When I went on the wards with the chief of the firm he asked me to stand some way away from the bedside, and then drew the curtains round the patient's bed - leaving me outside them. I could see nothing and I could hear very little of what was going on. I was left stranded in the middle of the ward with nothing to do but stand rather nervously by the nursing station, hoping that nobody would come and accost me, asking what I was doing there. It had been done without a word of explanation on the part of the physician, and I was worried that I had not made my wishes clear to him - that he was expecting this to be the regular pattern of my observations. After a quarter of an hour or so, the consultant and the students emerged from behind the screens and he explained to me that they had been examining a young woman with a difficult pregnancy. He had therefore not wanted to embarrass her with my presence. After that there was no question of my being excluded from his bedside teaching sessions, or those of his colleagues on the unit. Of course, given the nature of the work and teaching of general medicine and surgery, gynaecological examinations were not a regular part of the bedside instruction, and my presence was not normally a problem from that point of view.

My relations vis-à-vis patients raised other questions of ethics. It was generally a part of my negotiations for access that patients should be made aware of who I was and why I was present. This was a condition that I agreed to, as I had no wish to engage in more covert observation that I could avoid. However, in the event, my identity was never fully disclosed to any of the patients whom we went to see on the wards, and I was never explicitly introduced to them. As far as the patients were concerned, then, I was presumably a member of the student group, or another clinician, albeit a strangely silent one. When I joined students for their individual work with patients, they would often introduce me to the patient with some very vague phrase about my being there 'to see what we're doing', without indicating that I was not a regular member of the hospital or medical school. Members of staff never even volunteered such vague introductions.

To that extent, then, although I was an open observer with regard to the doctors and students, I was a disguised observer with regard to the patients. From my own point of view, this was less a deliberate research strategy, but more an exigency forced on me by the situation I was in. Control of teaching situations lay unequivocally with the teaching consultants, registrars or house officers. To that extent, both the negotiation of permission to teach, and disclosure of my identity, were the prerogative of the clinicians themselves. For me to attempt to enter into separate negotiations, and to achieve an open identity for myself when the clinicians remained silent, would have been to question the position of the doctors. It could have endangered the entire enterprise.

Just as I was a disguised observer vis-à-vis many of the patients, I was in a similar position with regard to the nursing and other para-medical staff. As I mingled with the various groups of students I passed as a student myself and I very rarely had occasion to negotiate a fresh identity with members of the nursing staff. The main occasion when I did so was on a surgical unit, when a theatre sister took an impromptu session with the students on basic surgical theatre technique (scrubbing up, putting on gloves and gowns). This fact is in itself telling: it highlights the degree of separation between the physicians and medical students on the one hand and the nursing staff on the other. There was little interaction between the two sides in the course of the clinical instruction I observed in two years of Medicine and Surgery. Rather, one's impression was one of a relatively self-contained group as clinician and students moved around the wards, insulated by a strong symbolic membrane. It was therefore, rather easy for me to have an open identity within a fairly limited group of people, and for me to pass as a taken-for-granted, socially invisible medical student.

The problem of disguised or secret observation has aroused considerable controversy in the literature of participant observation (Lofland and Lejeune, 1960; Davis, 1960; Roth, 1961; Humphreys, 1970). One aspect that has been raised in this context relates to the relative *power* of the researcher and the research hosts. The distribution of power and authority between the various parties was in great measure a determinant of my own position in the field. But the situation was not simply a reflection of my position vis-à-vis a single aggregate of actors. Most commentators imply that in one's field work, here is a *single* category of persons - the subjects with whom the fieldworker is either open or secret. For my part this was not the case. Not only was I concerned with staff, students and patients, but I was implicated in *their* power relationships. The power to grant or withhold the privilege of access to the group and its daily life was not equally shared by the students and the medical staff. It was quite possible for the staff to foist me onto their students, whilst the students had nothing like the same discretion in deciding whether I should observe their teachers. In the same way, I was very largely dependent on the doctors for my identity with the patients. It was very definitely the doctors who called the tune in that situation - for me, the students and the patients. Although the others had some leeway in redefining the situation, it was the doctor who routinely defined the task and who co-ordinated the activities of the actors. Had I made an issue of disclosure, then my position with the doctors would have been under threat.

Does the fact that the patient did not know who I was mean that I arrogated to myself some privileged status as a detached and uninvolved observer, above such personal and moral questions? I do not think so. On the contrary, I believe the reverse to be true. I believe that it was rather a recognition that I was on a par with the students and the other actors, and was myself implicated in their day-to-day interactions. Roth (1961) has a relevant comment here:

> When we are carrying out a piece of social research involving the behavior of other people, what do we tell them under what circumstances? Posing the question in this manner puts us in the same boat with physicians, social workers, prostitutes, policemen and others who must deal with information which is sometimes delicate,

threatening, and highly confidential. We are then in a position to draw upon our knowledge of these other groups and the way in which they handle information to carry out their work and to draw analogies between these professions and our own.

As I have tried to make clear, I was indeed 'in the same boat' with participants. There were many occasions and many patients when the doctors did not disclose information that they had access to: in some ways, my identity was one more piece of such information. In a study which addressed the control and exchange of information between students, patients and doctors, what the participants did or did not do with their knowledge of my identity was itself a very revealing source of insight into the dynamics of information-control at the bedside.

I am not trying to moralise on this point, and on the practices of the doctors concerned. The creation and maintenance of a bedside interaction is not a straightforward matter. The presence of students is itself a potentially threatening one. Their competence in clinical work and interactions cannot be assumed, and their participation is ambiguous, in that they are partly medical people and partly lay. The explicit addition of a totally lay person could have strained the encounter to an intolerable degree for the other participants. It is part of the price that we pay for undertaking naturalistic research that our fate in the field is very largely in the hands of others. The rhetoric of control is part of the language of experimental or quasi-experimental research: it is inherent in the method that the subjects of experimentation, and the setting of their behaviour should be under the control of the researcher to the maximum extent. In field work, such control has to be surrendered. The hosts are responsible for their own activities and for constituting the setting of the research. In my own field work I was to a great extent in the hands of the consultant doctors in matters of what I could and could not do, where I could go and so on. In this way, my relationship with the patients was almost entirely mediated by the acts of the doctors (and, occasionally, the students). My stance of closed or surreptitious observations of the patients was, therefore, not the result of my superior power, but a reflection of my inferior position. It must also be borne in mind that the status of the students was not always made clear to the patients. Sometimes doctors would introduce them as 'a group of medical students', sometimes as 'these young doctors'. To that extent, my own equivocal position was analogous to that of the students themselves.

Finally, it must also be added that in order to preserve the confidentiality of my observations, and the anonymity of the staff, students and patients concerned, all the names used in the course of writing the ethnography are pseudonyms. But I have not attempted to disguise the identity of all the hospitals involved - they are too well known in the context of the Edinburgh medical school for this to be realistic. However, there are occasions when the use of a particular hospital's name would limit reference to a single clinical unit, and hence by implication to a single chief of a firm. In such cases I have not referred to the hospital by name.

The researcher

It would be idle to pretend that the conduct of the research had no effect on me. On the contrary, it was a constant source of conflicting emotion. On the one hand, it provided areas of great personal satisfaction. On the other hand, it provided numerous occasions for embarrassment and anxiety. The personal nature of research of this sort means that fieldworkers cannot be seen as well-drilled automata. The conduct of participant observation requires considerable personal investment. The pay off on such an investment can be considerable, but the costs can be great as well. Fieldwork and participant observation can place considerable personal strain on researchers. It may require them to 'lay themselves on the line' in a number of potentially strange, difficult or embarrassing situations.

The disorientation experienced by social anthropologists in the field amongst alien cultures - the culture shock that they must undergo - is proverbial. Such social and personal isolation, coupled perhaps with physical discomfort, and even physical danger, is often seen as a necessary baptism of fire in which the novice anthropologist proves his mettle. For the sociologist engaged in research within striking distance of his or her own home territory the isolation may be less extreme, of shorter duration and more easily escapable. Nevertheless, while the observer is in play with the members of the community or organisation, he or she may also experience a degree of *Angst*. Although I was conducting my research on fellow members of my own University, I periodically found myself losing my nerve and having to force myself into the setting I wished to observe. At other times, although not faced with extreme emotional difficulty, I felt uneasy - out of things - and often heartily wished that I could 'cop out' of such research. The temptation to do the study by remote control - by anonymous postal questionnaires or library research - was often strong. I was frequently aware of my precarious position in the medical school. The teaching doctors had the power to order students to leave the wards if they were displeased with their appearance or behaviour, and their ability to do the same to me was perfectly obvious. Unlike the students, I could claim no legitimate 'medical' or educational reason for my presence.

In addition to general problems associated with the research approach I adopted, the subject matter under observation was also a potential source of personal response. I was by no means squeamish and I was able to accompany the students and surgeons and watch major operations without a qualm. Yet there were times when I was not so immune. On one occasion in a surgical unit I noted the following:

> Mr. Harrison led us out of the teaching room, saying that there was a patient on the ward, whose 'lesions' he thought that we would be 'interested' in seeing.
>
> I commented to two of the girls that I didn't think I really fancied looked at the lady's 'lesions': one of them replied that of course 'lesion' could mean anything down to a scratch on the nose.
>
> As it happened, my own worst fears were quite justified. Mr. Harrison took us across the landing to the procedure room by the men's ward. We all clustered behind a screen round a bed in the corner - it was quite a squeeze as we all shuffled round. The bed was occupied by a very fat woman, in middle age. Mr. Harrison said that he had brought some medical students to see her: it was quite clear that she didn't really have much choice in the matter, as we were all very much installed round her bed.
>
> The patient had dressings across her chest, and Mr. Harrison having gone to enlist the aid of a nurse, began to undo them. As he unwound the bandages, and removed the dressings, he uncovered the most appalling lesion that I have ever seen. I didn't look so closely that I could describe it at all accurately, but the woman's entire left breast appeared to have been eroded, and was the site of a ghastly mass of ulcerated and discoloured flesh. I was very grateful that I was at the back of the group and could keep the patient well out of my line of vision behind the backs and shoulders of some of the students.

Looking at their faces, I was quite surprised at their impassivity in the face of this frightful mess. I half expected that one of the girls might flake out, but apart from some very fixed looks, and some very pale faces, there was no observable untoward reaction. I could feel my own face going flushed.

My subsequent conversations with the students suggested that they too were all profoundly distressed by this particular case, just as I had been. There were also some distressing episodes in medical wards. On one attachment we paused on a ward-round to observe a house-physician who was already busy at a patient's bedside, preparing to take a sample of the patient's bone-marrow. Such samples are normally taken from the breast bone, but it was explained to us that a previous sample from that site had proved inadequate: it was not clear whether this arose from poor technique on the part of the physician who had carried out the procedure, or from a physiological cause. At any rate, it was now necessary to take a sample of marrow from the patient's iliac crest - in the pelvis. The procedure is carried out by boring a small core from the bone with a cork-screw-like instrument. The patient was an elderly woman. As we watched, the teaching clinician explained to us that it was not really possible completely to anaesthetise the bone against the procedure. We looked on as the houseman performed the procedure. As the young doctor bored into the patient's hip, and pulled out the plug of marrow, she screamed out in pain and cried out 'Mother, Oh, Mother!' On this and similar occasions I was very glad that - unlike the students - I was under no obligation to peer closely at what was going on. One or two of the students were very evidently distressed by the procedure, and one of the girls went very white and had to leave the bedside. She left the ward and went to sit down for a while to recover from her faintness. Although I was not an involved member of the group, I also felt somewhat shaken. Subsequently, the other students from the group reported that they too had felt distressed. Of course, such incidents were not the run-of-the-mill cases that we saw day in and day out on the wards. They were very much the exceptions. However, the awareness that such distressing episodes could take place also served to increase my feeling of insecurity on the wards.

In addition to such specific incidents, there were more general areas of discomfort. I certainly did not enjoy the few visits I made to the Acute Poisoning Unit - a forbidding ward, with little of the domestic bustle of the general wards, and one which dealt with a steady turnover of attempted suicides. The students and I were regularly depressed by our visits to this ward. Similarly, a visit to a hospital that housed long-term neurological patients was harrowing. As we left the ward for a mid-morning coffee-break on one such visit, one of the students exclaimed, 'Oh, God, preserve me from disseminated sclerosis!', and I concurred with him. It was far from pleasant to visit and talk to the patients with irreversible, degenerative disorders of the central nervous system. Their speech was affected, they were spastic, and presented a very sorry sight. In such surroundings it was impossible to switch off and act as if I were a detached observer.

In general, I felt more at home and more at ease on medical units than I did when on the surgical wards. I never felt entirely at ease with the post-operative paraphernalia of gastric tubes, drains and plastic bags that festooned some of the patients. Newly performed colostomies and ileostomies were relatively common, but were never pleasant.

Familiarity and learning

One of the methodological problems encountered in the course of the research arose by virtue of the social context of medicine. Medicine is an important and intrusive element in contemporary culture. A broad picture of what goes on in a hospital ward is part of the stock of knowledge which is possessed by every competent member of our culture. As Blanche Geer wrote in her classic discussion of the generation of problematics in the field:

> The concept of working hypothesis is not difficult, but field workers often have trouble explaining it to others and sometimes to themselves. The concept is clear, but its mechanics, the doing smacks of magic. *Untrained observers, for instance can spend a day in a hospital and come back with one page of notes and no hypotheses. It was a hospital, they say; everyone knows what hospitals are like.*
>
> (Geer, 1964. My emphasis)

When I began my research I was in no sense a 'trained observer' and although my first field notes were not as sparse as Geer suggests, I was certainly in some difficulty with much of the action that I observed. Although I was able to get some useful preliminary material from the various introductory lectures I attended with the students, when it came to my own observations of 'where the action was', I was much more at a loss. The problem initially resided in the *obviousness* and familiarity of the action scenes that I saw. The general features of the conduct of clinical medicine, and of clinical teaching are generally familiar. More or less colourful caricatures are available to many, if not all, members of our culture. As a reasonably well read and well informed layman, what I observed during my initial period in the field came as no great surprise. In Britain, such readily available portrayals of the conduct of clinical teaching are furnished by Richard Gordon's fictionalised account of life in a teaching hospital - particularly in the first volume of his saga - *Doctor in the House*. Although this book is explicitly humorous in intent, and it is drawn in somewhat exaggerated terms, *Doctor in the House* is based on first hand experience in a London teaching hospital, and it rings many bells with qualified doctors.

Becoming an expert

It is the task of the ethnographer to act as a self-conscious novice: to acquire knowledge of social organization and cultures whilst monitoring his or her own learning process:

> An observer, almost by definition, is one who does not understand. He is ignorant and needs to be taught. He has always to be watching and asking questions, whether his role as observer is known or unknown in a setting. In other words, he is a student. (Lofland, 1971, p.100)

In the course of my fieldwork in the medical school, I found myself needing to gain knowledge of two sorts. Both were varieties of inside knowledge in the medical school, and both constituted areas of learning for the students themselves. They could be referred to as organizational knowledge and technical knowledge respectively. Whilst the two intersect in many ways, I distinguish them here for analytic purposes.

The first type of knowledge that I refer to has been widely researched and commented on. It is the folk taxonomy of persons and occasions employed by groups. They are the everyday, practical ways in which workers classify their clients, their routine troubles and so on. These taxonomies are embodied in situated vocabularies (cf. Mills, 1940) which encapsulate members' typifications of their work situation - they are what Lofland (1971) calls 'member-identified types'. These types identify recurrent topics, tasks, objects or problems for the group members, and their invocation is normally accompanied by typical courses of action in perceiving, interacting or dealing with the designated persons or actions. Such a situated vocabulary has been identified in relation to medical students (Becker *et al.*, 1961, p.328) in their typifications of patients. The medical students at Kansas University recognise a type of patient whom they referred to as 'crocks' - a term used to 'refer to patients who disappoint them by failing to have pathological findings'. By contrast, although not specifically designated by any single term, the 'proper' patient was one who did have an identifiable (preferably treatable) illness. Manning (1971) suggests that the collection of such situated vocabularies constitutes a fundamental mode of data collection and analysis of socialisation processes. As novices are socialised into organisations, they acquire their sense of social structure, and of their position in it, through the medium of such typifications (cf. also Stoddart, 1974; Wieder, 1974).

An important focus of my own research in the Edinburgh Medical School was therefore attending to the recurrent vocabularies whereby the experience of clinical medicine was typified by the students and staff, and how the students used such categories in the course of generating and sharing their collective views of the medical school. The ways in which the students use some such typifications are presented elsewhere. Here I shall simply summarise the nature of the typifications that I discuss. Firstly, there were the ways in which the students came to categorise and characterise the various segments of the medical school - the academic and clinical subjects, the various teaching hospitals associated with the University, and the various clinical units in the hospitals. Closely related to these were the designations used by the students to describe their clinical teachers, and how they used their descriptive categories to produce types of doctors and their teaching. Thirdly, I paid attention to how the students themselves classified the *times* and *places* within which teaching (or other activities) took place. The students would classify occasions, and had notions which implied what might legitimately be expected to happen at different times and in different milieux. Clearly, like Becker's students at Kansas, the Edinburgh students might be expected to hold views on categories of patients, and to employ their own taxonomies of such highly relevant others. During my field research, then, I was on the lookout for the development and use of such patient-designations as part of the students' perspectives on their clinical work.

The recording of such members' vocabularies is clearly an important part of any field-researcher's task. The process of becoming competent in the daily lives of the members of a group necessarily involves the mastery of such folk-systems. The development of such comprehension is a vital aspect of the researcher's own acquisition of a sense of social reality, as it is constructed and construed by the group whose life he shares.

This aspect of 'inside' knowledge is not necessarily the only one which may be involved in the activities that are observed, and in which the researcher participates. In addition to the folk-types that members use, there may also be esoteric and specialised knowledge which is the preserve of an epistemic collectivity, such as a profession. Specialist knowledge of various sorts is the stock-in-trade of most occupational groups, and the question arises of the extent to which one needs to master aspects of this expertise in order to conduct research on the occupational group. This problem has not been adequately discussed by writers on field work methods. It appears to be taken for granted that such knowledge is not the proper concern for sociological investigation. Yet it is an extremely important topic and resource for the community members themselves. It may be the subject of discussion, of difference of opinion and so on amongst the experts. In the course of their day-to-day work, the members of the epistemic community draw upon their expertise in the actual performance of their daily tasks, and in arriving at decisions about their work.

It may, therefore, be of importance, that the ethnographer gain some acquaintance with the esoteric knowledge of the group or occupation under observation. A concern for the management of knowledge in educational settings as a topic for field research imposes on the ethnographer the requirement of at least some acquaintance with the group's specialist knowledge. In the context of my own research, this was not too difficult. The events that I was witnessing and participating in were explicitly defined as *teaching* episodes; the students themselves were being taught the knowledge which formed much of the content of the interaction. Although I did not possess any special grounding in the medical sciences, I too found that I was being 'taught' medicine - vicariously, as it were, through my participation with the medical students. Bedside teaching is an extremely vivid form of teaching; 'real' patients provide very memorable 'audio-visual' aids in teaching. Willy-nilly, I picked up a great deal of *ad hoc* medical information, and some rudimentary expertise in clinical medicine and surgery. I also made reference to text-books, such as Davidson's *Principles and Practice of Medicine* (written by members of the Edinburgh medical school staff) to check up on cases that I had seen on the wards during the day.

The students often found it hard to believe that I was genuinely capable of understanding what was going on - and on occasion would commiserate with me on my 'obvious' inability to follow what I was observing. They sometimes seemed unable or unwilling to believe that I was indeed able to keep up with at least the greater part of what was going on. Some students even appeared to resent my ability to gain some passing acquaintance with their subject, without the background training in the basic and medical sciences. However, much of what the students were taught was translated into everyday terminology; also, much of the clinical methodology that they were taught was directly based upon mundane powers of observation and reasoning, and as such, it was accessible to anybody who had privileged' access to the teaching occasion. Whilst diagnostic inferences may be based partly on knowledge of physiology, anatomy and biochemistry, the observation of patients' complexion and general physical appearance, their gait and other behaviour do not normally depend upon any such esoteric knowledge on the students' part.

The topic that I am considering here can be seen as one concerned with the social distribution of knowledge in the field. In developing it further I shall begin by outlining Schutz's characterisation of ideal-types of knowledge, and their associated roles. Schutz (1964) distinguishes in people's repertoires of knowledge about the world, three types of knowledge. In the first place, there are areas where we have 'explicit knowledge of *what* is aimed at'. Secondly, there are areas where we have 'knowledge *about* what seems to be sufficient'. Thirdly, there 'comes a region in which it will do merely "to put one's trust"'. These varieties will be related to the degrees of relevance to the actor in her or his daily life - there will be ranges of topics in which he needs a close and detailed knowledge, and ranges where a 'nodding acquaintance' is sufficient for his normal practical interests. Schutz uses this notion to develop an ideal-typical formulation of three social types associated with three varieties of knowledge (Schutz, 1964, p.93ff). From the point of view of any particular given activity or interest, we can distinguish 'the expert', 'the well-informed citizen' and 'the man-on-the-street'. Schutz (1964, pp. 121-123) describes these types in the following terms:

> The expert's knowledge is restricted to a limited field but therein it is clear and distinct. His opinions are based upon warranted assertions; his judgements are not mere guesswork or loose suppositions.
> The man on the street has a working knowledge of many fields which are not necessarily coherent with one another. His is a knowledge of recipes indicating how to bring forth in typical situations typical results by typical means. The

recipes indicate procedures which can be trusted even though they are not clearly understood. By following the prescription as if it were a ritual the desired result can be attained without questioning why the single procedural steps have to be taken and taken exactly in the sequence prescribed. This knowledge in all vagueness is still *sufficiently* precise for the practical purpose at hand. In all matters not connected with such practical purposes of immediate concern the man on the street accepts his sentiments and passions as guides. Under their influence, he establishes a set of convictions and unclassified views which he simply relies upon as long as they do not interfere with his pursuit of happiness.

The ideal type that we propose to call the well-informed citizen (thus shortening the more correct expression: the citizen who aims at being well informed) stands between the ideal type of the expert and that of the man on the street. On the one hand, he neither is, nor aims at being, possessed of expert knowledge; on the other hand he does not acquiesce in the fundamental vagueness of a mere recipe knowledge or in the irrationality of his unclarified passions and sentiments. To be well informed means to me to arrive at *reasonably* founded opinions in fields which as he knows are at least mediately of concern to him although not bearing upon his purpose at hand.

On entry to the field, while familiar with the general nature of hospital life, I was certainly a 'man in the street' when it came to the technical vocabulary and knowledge of clinical medicine. However, in the course of doing the research I found myself becoming a 'well informed citizen'. To some extent I cultivated basic medical knowledge as a resource in doing the research. I did try to make a point of noting and, if necessary, looking up technical terms in medicine and surgery. This was a personal reward for the conduct of the research - a personal satisfaction gained in the acquisition of such knowledge. I also found it necessary to note some of the technical detail. For example, it might happen that there was disagreement over the diagnosis of a patient between the doctors who taught the students; or, in the course of time, the diagnosis would be changed. In following such developments, some attention to the technical detail of the doctors' and students' talk provided me with benchmarks in charting these shifts of definition and in the comparison of the divergent opinions. It is always difficult to follow prolonged discussions on topics which are mostly alien and poorly understood. Not only do the nuances and details of such talk get overlooked, but also major topics of discussion may otherwise pass over the observer's head. The topic of pharmacology was an area in which I found it particularly expedient to develop some acquaintance with specialist medical knowledge - primarily a grasp of the range of generic and proprietary names of drugs that were most commonly referred to. This did not mean that I was tempted to become an expert in the various specialist subjects. In recording my notes, I was not concerned with evaluating whether the students were 'right' or 'wrong' in their replies to doctors' questions. Nor was I worried about whether what the doctors told their students was in accord with contemporary scientific orthodoxy. Thus I did not need to learn the precise metabolic action of the drugs and so attempt to become an expert on pharmacology and biochemistry (even if I had been capable of such a task). However, the ability to recognise and make some clinical sense of the topics of teaching sessions did enable me to produce much more detailed and faithful field notes than would otherwise have been possible. It will be apparent throughout the thesis that my notes often contain a good deal of clinical terminology, and I have done my best to make its meaning clear.

What I am suggesting is that while there is no necessity for a fieldworker to become an 'expert' in medicine (or whatever), it may be advantageous to become something of a 'well informed citizen' in performing the research. In the context of my own research, the fact that I was observing educational occasions made the acquisition of such knowledge fairly straight-forward. There were many areas of clinical work which were novel to the students themselves, and had to be explained to them by the clinicians. In the course of such educational talk, things were made more explicit to the students, and spelled out in some detail; hence I often found that by following the content of tutorials or bedside teaching sessions I also picked up the same basic clinical knowledge. In this respect, educational situations may be easier to follow than those involving only qualified and competent members of an occupation, when more things might be taken for granted and passed over without explanation. Learners can provide vicarious experiences of learning for the ethnographer, while the ethnographer learns from instructional talk and action.

I did, of course, use my genuine ignorance as a research resource. The fact that I was not medically qualified meant that I could repeatedly (and often disingenuously) plead ignorance or a lack of understanding.

Such appeals to my status as a naive outsider permitted me to ask for clarification of points and accounts of activities which might otherwise have come oddly from an expert in the field. As Lofland points out, it is often expedient to act in such a way as to portray oneself as an 'ignorant-student-who-has-to-be-taught', and to make a virtue of one's ignorance. On the basis of such 'ignorance' one may legitimately ask the questions by which 'what everyone knows' must be made explicit by the members concerned (Lofland, 1971). As Lofland says, 'there may ... be a split between being an acceptable incompetent and needing to be an insider expert'. I found it necessary to manage the contrasting impressions of both expertise and ignorance in the course of my fieldwork in the medical school. My general point here is to emphasise that the methodological stance of outsider, novice or stranger does not absolve the ethnographer from the requirement to make sense of the esoteric knowledge of a given community or occupation. One cannot make serious sociological sense of medical knowledge and medical culture if one remains stubbornly ignorant of what medical practitioners and their students actually do (Atkinson, 1984).

Methodological retrospect

At the time when I conducted the research for the thesis, and its subsequent publication, there were remarkably few methodological models and textbooks available. A small number of texts, such as those by Lofland or Schatzman and Strauss, an equally small number of edited collections, and the oral traditions in anthropology and sociology were among the very sparse sources of advice and legitimation. The contrast between the early 1970s, when I did the fieldwork, and the preparation of new edition is stark. In comparison, the extent of methodological advice has expanded beyond all recognition. If anything, there is now probably too much methodological literature, and today's aspiring student could easily drown in the volume of precepts and exemplars. I have not attempted to doctor this chapter in order to convey a spurious air of contemporary sophistication. It reflects, rather, how the research was actually conducted and understood. I have contented myself with providing a much fuller account of the research than was available previously.

There have, of course, been significant changes in the discipline that impinge on the conceptualization and conduct of ethnographic work. Not least has been the increase in techniques of data collection and analysis.

There have, indeed, been repeated attempts to typologise the varieties of qualitative research method. In the contemporary intellectual climate one cannot escape the sense that ethnographic fieldwork is a more complicated business than it was when I did the Edinburgh study. There appear to be multiple decisions and choices to be made, with multiple analytic consequences. To a considerable extent, however, I suspect that many of these reflect the pedagogical discriminations of the classroom and the textbook, rather than the contingencies of fieldwork in practice. That may be true even of the introduction of computer-aided qualitative data analysis since the completion of this research. As I have argued elsewhere (Weaver and Atkinson 1994; Coffey, Holbrook and Atkinson 1996), the vast majority of uses of qualitative data analysis software do little to transform the intellectual processes of data analysis. They seem to recapitulate the kinds of 'manual' procedures of data management that were characteristic of my original research project. In the absence of text-files on a PC, my data were managed as hard copy (mostly hand-written processed fieldnotes), marked up with a restricted set of analytic themes. While the mechanics of data management and analysis might have been improved upon by the use of computer software, in retrospect I am not convinced that the overall thrust of my treatment of the research setting would have been very different. The more explicit mechanisms of coding and retrieving data segments might have made for a more densely coded data set, and more systematic, comprehensive searching of those data. Nevertheless, the general approach of the analysis would probably have been similar. Indeed, as I explore in one of the new sections of this edition, a retrospective view of the original analysis suggests that the computer-aided approaches I have been referring to would have encouraged and confirmed the original approach, rather than suggesting radically alternative perspectives on the data.

4 Counting experience and organizing careers

Judging cliniques

In the course of their clinical year the students have an interest in the accumulation of 'clinical experience', and in the organisation of their student careers. For most of them this is the first time when they exercise choice in charting a personal course through the medical school. For each of the three terms of the year students are asked to state their preference as to which clinic they should like to attend. Although it does not guarantee attachment to a particular unit, a student's choice does significantly affect the chances of a placement, and hence the nature of the clinical experience he or she amasses.

Each of the clinical units available in medicine and surgery enjoys a high degree of autonomy with regard to the provision made for undergraduate teaching. Each clinical unit develops its own arrangements, which reflect the clinical and educational commitments of the staff members involved. Each unit can, in theory at least, offer the student a unique educational experience. It is therefore, an important part of the 'art and practice of studentship' (Olesen and Whittaker, 1968) that students should attempt to acquire and use information which they believe to be relevant to their choices between the various medical and surgical cliniques. On the basis of such information, they need to plan an undergraduate career which best satisfies their personal plans.

This interest is a major preoccupation of the local student culture. Becker and Geer (1960) describe such culture in this way:

> This culture grows around those problems shared by all students in the school, problems related to their manifest identities as students; the immediate necessity of mastering a vast amount of factual material, the more distant threat of failing, the difficulties of dealing with details of work in

the hospital, and the peculiarities of certain teachers and departments.

Such remarks apply equally well to the recurrent preoccupations and problems of the Edinburgh students. The choice and 'evaluation' of clinical units is almost exclusively a matter of student culture, and is all but totally based on information shared within the student body. (One or two students from Edinburgh medical families have additional sources of information: they can obtain inside knowledge which otherwise is usually unavailable.)

At the outset, of course, the fourth-year students all lack firsthand experience of any clinical units. In order to acquire reliable 'tips', they must look to those who have already been through that part of the course, and who therefore 'know the ropes' (cf. Geer *et al.* 1968). They look to students in the fifth and sixth years to advise them on the best course of action, and as to the relevant criteria in judging units and evaluating their educational experience. In this way the accumulated folk wisdom of the student culture is passed on from cohort to cohort.

As the year unfolds the fourth years begin to have their own experiences to exchange. Indeed, from the very first day on the wards, they enthusiastically swap anecdotes and evaluations about their patients, their teachers and the organisation of their clinical work. As they meet informally after teaching, the students compare notes about their own progress, and about the qualities of their respective cliniques. The students are thus engaged, at an informal level, in a process of 'continuous assessment' of their teachers and teaching.

This is not to imply that there is complete consensus within the student culture. Some cliniques are almost universally approved of: other are pretty well unanimously regarded as poor. But there are many instances where opinions differ as to the relative merits of different clinical units. For the student seeking advice it is often a matter of 'you pays your money and you takes your choice'. The students recognise that the whole process can be something of a lottery. Some indeed opt out of the business of information seeking and sharing: they pick their attachments more or less at random.

Collectively, then, the students are actively engaged in monitoring the educational experience offered in the various cliniques. Individually, they plan their passage through their various attachments, and evaluate them as they progress. They judge what they refer to as the 'atmosphere' of cliniques, a general student term which embraces a number of evaluative criteria.

In organising their evaluations of different clinical units, the students use a sort of folk taxonomy (cf. Atkinson, 1977). The major discrimination which students use to differentiate cliniques is unsurprisingly, the contrast between Medicine and Surgery. Throughout the year they draw parallels and contrasts between the two specialties. In addition, they divide the teaching hospitals into two types: 'central' and 'peripheral'. In the broader context this latter pair of terms is a relative one: a hospital which is regarded as central from one point of view may be seen as peripheral from another. Thus in comparison with hospitals in outlying areas all the Edinburgh hospitals may be called central. But when they differentiate between the Edinburgh hospitals, students refer to the Royal Infirmary as the centre, and to the other teaching hospitals as peripheral. A further distinction is drawn between professorial and non-professorial units. In the former, the clinical staff are University employees, and the firm is headed by a professor; the staff hold honorary NHS appointments. The non-professional units are staffed by NHS clinicians, who may hold honorary University posts.

The students use these dimensions to generate their own map of the relevant portions of the medical school. While the categories of unit are based on aspects of the formal organisation of the school and the hospitals, the students endow them with their own, informal, connotations. It is believed that while each clinic has its own unique atmosphere, they vary systematically in line with these dimensions. The students offer each other generalisations: 'all surgical units are ...'; 'peripheral hospitals tend to ...'; 'you'll find that the professorial cliniques are more ...'. On the basis of such typifications students seek out likely cliniques for their own training. They also attempt to relate the typical expectations of the student culture to their own past and present experiences of individual cliniques.

Staff and students

As in other educational milieux, their relationships with staff members is an important element in the students' evaluations of clinic atmosphere. For these junior students, their working relations with clinical staff, especially consultants, are of particular moment, and are potentially fraught. In the first place, the clinical teachers are themselves practitioners, and are potential superiors in students' subsequent work. Even if individual members of staff are not seen as likely hirers and firers, students are keenly aware of the professional hierarchy. (Some individual consultants, of course, may stand very high in the medical pantheon.) Similarly, the reality-like nature of clinical instruction means that the teacher student relationship is a key element in the students' experience of clinical work and clinical instruction. All in all, consultants in medicine and surgery in the teaching hospitals may present a daunting prospect for young novices.

The clinical teaching often takes place in a charged atmosphere. The small-group teaching sessions can be quite demanding on the students. They are in play for the duration of the teaching, and may be called on to perform before their peers, the clinician and the patient, in taking a history and performing an examination. The students may be grilled on their medical knowledge, also in this semi-public fashion. While one should not over dramatise the extent to which the students are on trial, it does give an edge to their day to day relations with clinicians, particularly with the more senior staff members.

For these junior students, the exposure to clinical medicine, real patients and clinical teachers, is a potentially threatening experience. The atmosphere which is created and sustained on a clinical unit is therefore a critical consideration for them. It is possible for clinicians to make life extremely uncomfortable for students. They have available to them, for instance, the technique of 'showing them up' (Woods, 1985) before the patients and their peers. As Wood shows, in a very different educational context, students are vulnerable to the weapons of sarcasm, humiliation and degradation. To give just one extreme example: I observed one rather irascible consultant physician respond in this way to a student he regarded as having performed ineptly:

> 'What's your name?'
> 'Reid, sir'.
> 'And where do *reeds* grow? In dark wet places - you idiot!'

(I have changed the student's name in such a way as to preserve the force of the consultant's vicious pun.) Such extreme tongue lashings are, of course, rare, and seldom so venomous. But students are frequently, and understandably, reluctant to show themselves up, or to be shown up. Bedside interaction, then, can be tense for the potentially incompetent student (cf. Haas and Shaffir, 1977; DelVecchio Good, 1995). In the clinical setting the medical student's identity and self-esteem are constantly open to threat and damage. Each patient and each clinician can make demands that exceed the student's knowledge or skills. The Socratic dialogue through which much medical instruction takes place repeatedly singles out individual students for cross-examination. His or her peers provide the audience when the student is thus 'shown up'.

Students are also concerned with their incorporation and involvement into the 'team' of clinical staff on the wards. On entering the first clinical year, the students have crossed a major divide in their careers, and have, in some degree, entered the real world of clinical hospital medicine. In the course of their clinical instruction, the students' perspective is that of the doctors, rather than that of other health workers on the ward. Yet the students are not doctors themselves. They do not perform the same tasks, do not have comparable responsibilities, functions or status. Their position is therefore an ambiguous one, poised somewhat uncertainly between the lay world and the medical world of their teachers. Their involvement in the wards is only temporary and part-time; they are subordinate and marginal. Yet, for the most part, they would like to be made to feel a part of things. Hence the precise nature of students' relations with their clinical instructors can assume a critical significance in the development of their self-perceptions and their evaluation of clinical atmosphere.

The fourth-year students therefore pay close attention to their position vis-a-vis the doctors on their attachments. There are two related issues. The first concerns the degree of personal contact between clinicians and students. Despite the students' close proximity to the clinicians, the actual teaching can come over as anonymous and impersonal. Especially in units where a large number of doctors have teaching responsibilities, students may find that they remain unknown as individuals. The learning of their names by staff, for instance, is one indicator used to gauge the staff's interest in students and the degree of colleagueship that is established. For example, in characterising a surgical unit as unfavourable, one student remarked, 'Mr.Williams is the only one who's bothered to learn names'; by contrast, the feeling (rightly or wrongly) was that the other surgeons had not bothered to identify the students as individuals.

As this suggests, the students also attempt to judge the staff members' interest in teaching them. They recognise that clinical teaching is only one of a number of calls on a physician's or a surgeon's time - including routine patient care, research and administration. They appreciate the competing demands on their time and energy. They are mindful too that for junior staff there may be the pressure of their own training and work for Fellowship or Membership examinations (for the Royal College of Surgeons and Physicians respectively). But they get the impression that the degree of commitment displayed towards the teaching of fourth years

71

varies considerably from doctor to doctor, and from unit to unit. For instance:

> Jane told me she had applied to a surgical firm: but she had been down there with Frances (her flatmate and another fourth year medical student) to see one of the surgeons there. He had said, 'Oh, do we have to do all that teaching again?' She obviously took this to indicate a lack of interest in the teaching programme. She added that she understood surgeons had been telling the students to go away and read things up in the Medical Reading Room, rather than teaching them.

Students therefore employ this criterion in categorising clinic atmosphere. For instance, I asked one student what sort of thing he went on in choosing cliniques:

> Well, the report of the teaching, and sort of how organised it is and how interested they seem in teaching the students. 'Cos I mean some units, they don't - they'd rather get on with hard work rather than teach students, and in others they're very pleased to see you. Teaching is something they quite enjoy, probably because it provides them with a bit of amusement as well when you do something wrong.

This evaluation is often used to discriminate between medicine and surgery. It is a frequently voiced typification that the surgeons often appear 'uninterested' or 'uninvolved' in their work with the junior students. For example, as students told me:

> Both medicine wards have been very good though emotionally traumatic. Surgery was poor - the staff seemed very uninterested.
> On [surgical unit] I don't think I really got to know the staff, or that they took very much interest in us, in comparison with the last place [a medical unit].

The nature of staff-student relationships is also used to distinguish between units in the 'centre' and in the 'periphery'. The clinical teachers at 'the Royal' are thought, on the whole, to expect a greater degree of formality and to encourage a greater social distance between themselves and the students. Clinicians in other hospitals (especially physicians) are thought to foster a much more 'relaxed' atmosphere.

The degree of 'friendliness' and 'colleagueship' which students feel in their relations with clinicians is also felt to be a reflection of the quality of working relationships between the ward professionals themselves. The central units of the Royal Infirmary are believed to have a particularly competitive ethos. Although the students report that they enjoy good relationships with junior staff in The Royal, they also feel that these younger physicians and surgeons are acutely aware of their own career contingencies. The Infirmary is seen as that part of the medical school which enjoys the highest prestige, thus recruiting the ablest and most ambitious young men and women (though there are few enough of the latter). The students therefore feel that these junior doctors are involved in a 'rat-race' (as many of them phrased it), competing for recognition, jealous of each other's research productivity, and jostling for the consultant's attention. Whether or not the students are correct in thinking that this is particularly acute in the Infirmary, it is certainly the case that generally there is a great deal of competition for promotion in such popular hospital specialties as medicine and surgery.

Competition is also felt to characterise the professional relationships of the more senior staff members. It is argued that in the 'peripheral' hospitals, the consultant staff enjoy friendly relations, whereas this intimacy is lacking in the more formal atmosphere of the Royal Infirmary. At the same time the consultants at 'the Royal' are thought to compete with each other, in terms of their professional standing, their expertise, and the treatment of esoteric conditions. (I have no direct information on the actual quality of professional relations. But it must be pointed out that the Infirmary is a good deal larger and more complex organisation than the so-called peripheral hospitals, where greater intimacy may be more readily achieved.)

Although relationships among the staff do not normally impinge directly on the fourth-year students, the students themselves take this aspect of ward life as a reflection of the more general and pervasive ethos of a given clinical unit. Indeed, this atmosphere is felt to colour the attitudes of nursing staff. Admittedly, the junior students do not have all that much direct contact with the nurses. But they do form impressions of the nurses' attitudes towards students. For instance, they judge whether the nurses regard students as an unwelcome intrusion on the wards (or at least whether they convey such reservations by word or deed).

In all these ways, then, the fourth year students attempt to make sense of their introduction to the hospital wards, and to judge the extent to which they are granted some degree of colleagueship by their clinical teachers. These concerns are parallelled by comparable interests in their relations with the hospital patients.

Relations with patients

For the fourth-year students it is the outstanding feature of their introduction to clinical work that they begin to work with actual patients. Such patient contact is the touchstone of the authenticity of their medical experience. It is also crucial to their own developing self-perception as young doctors in the making. At the same time they are concerned to monitor not only their own interaction with patients, but also those of their teachers (cf. Dowling and Cotsonas, 1964). Specifically, they try to assess whether the hospital doctors deal with their patients in a considerate and humane fashion.

There has been a long-standing interest in the 'idealism' or 'cynicism' of medical students and other professionals in training. One version of the argument suggests that students begin with a predisposition towards idealism: in the course of their professional training, that character trait is gradually replaced by one of cynicism (e.g. Eron, 1955). An alternative view suggests that this apparent change is not a matter of psychological characteristics. Rather, it is seen as a reflection of *situational* factors. That is, a display of 'cynicism', or something like it, is a part of medical school culture: it is the 'done thing' to express such attitudes, at least in public, this latter view proposes, but that does not necessarily reveal fundamental changes in attitude (e.g. Becker and Geer, 1958).

That argument is primarily one about socialisation, about the effect of medical school over time. It is, of course, more than that: it reflects competing theories and methodologies, as well as honest-to-goodness conceptual muddle. In the nature of things the research reported here cannot deal with such change directly. It was, however, noticeable that the students did employ notions which might be called 'idealistic' (though one of the conceptual problems I referred to is the fact that 'idealism' and 'cynicism' gloss over a legion of possible attitudes, vocabularies of motive and so on). The fourth-year students recognise that in order to survive as a medical student, one had to 'harden' oneself; that it would be no use to be squeamish or emotionally vulnerable. Nevertheless they expect to be able to establish sympathetic relationships with their patients, and to preserve a degree of what Lief and Fox (1963) call 'detached concern'. They expect their clinical teachers to display the same concern, and they judge them accordingly. They do not find that the doctors are all equally 'humane' in their approach (or at least, do not appear to be so).

Among other things, the students use this criterion to distinguish between the typical features of their experiences in medicine and surgery. It is a commonly voiced criticism of surgery that the observed relationships between the surgeons and their patients are not as satisfying as those pertaining between the physicians and their patients. The surgeons appear to place much less emphasis on the interpersonal aspects of their patient care.

According to this view, the surgeons come over to their students as more 'callous', 'brusque' or 'offhand' with their patients. They seem to approach their work with a much more limited focus than do the physicians. They are often seen as concentrating more on the purely physical aspects of patient care - concerned with the technicalities of surgery itself - than on the care and well-being of the 'whole patient'. Students hold up the ideal of treating each patient individually, as a 'person' rather than as a 'case', and the majority find the surgeons lacking. (As is usually the case with such stereotyping, the student view does not explicate what would *actually* be implied by 'treating patients as people'.) Some students argue vigorously on the surgeons' behalf, maintaining that the stereotype is false - that surgeons are not really callous, and practise a type of medicine every bit as good as that practised by the physicians. Yet even these defenders acknowledge the potency of the negative stereotype among their classmates. Certainly the detractors of surgery are in the majority. Rightly or wrongly, they voice the criticism that the surgeons tend to see patients primarily as 'a lump' or 'a stomach' rather than as 'Mr or Mrs So-and-So'. As an indicator of this attitude, the students claim to observe that surgeons remember their patients' names less often than do the physicians.

This criterion is also drawn on in the students' comparison of central and peripheral units. The more 'impersonal' atmosphere which they associate with 'the Royal' is felt to colour doctor patient relationships. The students' folk wisdom has it that, for both medicine and surgery, the peripheral units tend towards a more 'patient centred' approach to practice. The 'central' firms, on the other hand, are held to exemplify a contrasting medical ideology. The doctors on such units are generally believed to concentrate their efforts on more technological or scientific styles, at the expense of patient oriented medicine. They are said to be more interested in academic, research oriented work.

The students' expectations and perceptions of their own patient contacts mirror their ideas about doctor-patient relationships. There is a sharp difference between medicine and surgery. In keeping with the views outlined above, the students' experience is that they themselves are able to form more and closer relations with patients on the medical wards than they are in surgery. As I have already indicated, the opportunity to work with patients on the ward is an especially salient feature of the students' experience, and the opportunity to engage in such clinical work is highly valued. Consequently, the fourth year students judge the various clinical firms in terms of the scope they offer for working directly with patients, and thus of accumulating personal experience of something they regard as central to 'real' clinical medicine.

Most medical units are felt to offer adequate opportunity for such experience to be acquired. A relatively high proportion of the time is spent in bedside teaching, and there is correspondingly less emphasis on tutorials or lectures in the unit's teaching rooms. While attached to medical wards, therefore, students are able to feel that they spend more of their time at the 'coal face' of clinical practice. At this early stage in the clinical phase of their undergraduate training, it is understandable that work with patients should have such a high value, if only in terms of novelty - in addition to its value in symbolising authentic medicine. The chance to clerk patients is probably the most highly prized clinical opportunity of this sort. Students can then work with an individual patient over a more protracted period than is usually possible, often spread over several days. Working alone, taking a full history and completing a thorough physical examination, they can sometimes develop the valued rapport with a patient. Moreover, this exercise approximates most closely the actual clinical work performed by the doctors. Students are normally expected to write up their cases, outlining the main findings, and essaying differential diagnosis. Such a product, the case notes, is tangible evidence of the real clinical work the students put in, and its production mimics the actual work put in by the medical staff on admitting a patient.

The students' initial experience of such clinical matters (gained on medical units in the first term of the year) is treasured as a major step forward in their accumulation of relevant experience. When they progress to a surgical attachment in the second or third term, they often find themselves disappointed. There is, they report, less scope for such contact with patients. There is, in the first place, more emphasis on lectures or seminars, less on bedside teaching and ward rounds. Secondly, there is less opportunity to clerk patients and follow through individual cases. Consequently, the students tend to evaluate surgical units negatively and to compare them unfavourably with their medical attachments. They grumble that they lack sufficient contact with the patients, have little chance to take a detailed case history or perform a systematic physical examination. They complain too that while they are on a surgical wards they have insufficient time to practise their new clinical skills. The techniques which have been so dearly acquired during their introductory week are, they maintain, 'getting rusty'. Furthermore, this lack of patient contact robs the students of opportunities to experience their emerging identities as young doctors in the context of real patient care.

Detective work

There is one aspect of clinical work which the students appreciate in particular. They often refer to it as 'detective work'. The task of history-taking, physical examination and differential diagnosis presents the students with something which is, potentially, a satisfying and stimulating intellectual exercise. Thus students learn to spot the distinctive, pathognomic indications of particular diseases, and the skills necessary to elicit relevant clinical information. Their clinical teachers encourage the use of the 'special senses', exhorting the students to use their powers of observation and inference to the full. Occasionally, they are encouraged to make an 'end-of-the bed' spot diagnosis on the basis of some readily observable clinical sign. On other occasions, the students need to piece together more complex information, perhaps called from different sources (the clinical findings, test results, X-ray plates and the like). However it is done, this process of diagnosis is highly valued and success at it is a source of some pride.

This sort of inquiry and reasoning is associated particularly with internal medicine, which is therefore seen as a more enjoyable and absorbing enterprise: the concerns of surgery, on the other hand, are seen to be much more limited - the surgeons' work being more restricted in intellectual and practical scope. Many of the students formulate a stereotype in which the surgeon's diagnostic task is less demanding than the physician's. He (rarely she) may have to be no more precise than to identify an 'acute abdomen', and then 'go in' and 'have a look'. The surgeon can deal directly with the patient's condition, whereas the physician has to work at a distance. Where the physician has to rely on clinical inference, the surgeon can, in the last resort, confirm a diagnostic hunch by direct observation. As one student put it:

Surgery is very limited intellectually. You can make a diagnosis, but it's not so crucially important because in the end you're going to cut the patient up anyway, and find out whether you're right or wrong.

At their least charitable the students claim that the surgeon is more of a technician or craftsman ('a carpenter' is a frequent epithet), seen as a manual worker, as opposed to the more cerebral physician. Similarly, surgeons are said to work mainly on rather specific, localised disease (a fact which contributes to their treatment of patients as 'cases'). The problems of internal medicine are often more general and more diffuse, making greater demands on the physicians' clinical acumen.

It probably goes without saying that this view of surgery is not one with which most surgeons would agree, and it is not the image which they consciously project for the specialty in their teaching. There is a small minority of students who do not subscribe to the popular stereotype: they find in surgery intellectual challenge and satisfaction, and defend the specialty against the detractors. In particular they take issue with the belief that surgery is limited intellectually, and point out the complexities of post operative care, as well as the sheer technical expertise involved in its practice.

It might be thought that surgery would offer its own compensating advantages to the fourth year students. Generally speaking, surgery has a glamour all of its own - not least, in the popular view of this branch of medicine. One might reasonably expect the fourth year students to be pleased and even enthusiastic at the idea of direct exposure to surgical operations. To some extent this is the case. Certainly at the very outset the students do appreciate the change to observe the surgeons at work in the theatre. As with other aspects of clinical work, students gain the impression that they are participating in the 'reality' of hospital medicine. The first operations which students observe are treated as landmarks in their growing clinical experience. But for many of them the novelty soon wears off. The reason for this is not hard to find. As very junior novices, the students' role in surgery must always be that of passive observers of the scene rather than that of active participants. For the most part, there is little for a group of up to twelve students to do other than watch an operation from an observation gallery. Ultimately, then, the students' distance from and lack of involvement in the surgical work is emphasised. Their junior status is reinforced, and they rarely feel incorporated as junior colleagues. Occasional visits to the operating theatre gallery are, as

I have suggested, occasions for the display of clinical spectacle. Paradoxically, however, they emphasise the extent to which the students are *audience*. The surgeon's dominant position as the centre of the action and the accompanying commentary contrasts with the passivity of the students and their lack of intellectual engagement. A considerable proportion find the experience disappointingly marginalising: it stands in sharp contrast to popular imagery and students' own reported expectations concerning excitement and engagement.

Waiting nights, on the other hand, do provide some opportunity for students to gain experience of more direct involvement. Since they normally attend in small numbers (usually a couple at a time) it is much more feasible for the fourth year students to become more involved with the work of the surgeons. They can see patients admitted, and are often able to follow them through into theatre. At such times the one or two fourth years present have a much better chance of observing the surgery at close quarters. If they are lucky they also get the chance to assist at operations (in practice, something like holding a retractor). This sort of participation is viewed very positively. But such occasions tend to be rare 'treats', in comparison with routine instruction in surgery.

Students prize operations that they have observed at close hand or at which they have assisted. Be they only minor operations - for haemorrhoids, or a circumcision, say - the first few are highly significant benchmarks in the collection of clinical experience. They are recounted by students to their friends, with not a little personal pride. (Obviously this only works during these early days of clinical training. Later in their careers they would hardly be able to boast of having been present at a circumcision.)

One of the central surgical units I observed has an arrangement whereby a small group of students in the clinique can attend a small peripheral hospital for part of their attachment. There it is possible for them to be more directly involved in the day to day work of the surgeons. There is a remarkable contrast between the students' enthusiasm for this brief period of their work and their relative indifference towards their work on the 'proper' unit. They are eager to recount their experiences in the periphery, and to catalogue the operations (not in themselves very serious or dramatic) which they had closely observed or assisted at. Their experience serves to highlight that of the majority of students who do not have an equivalent opportunity.

Work and effort

The likely level of effort in different firms is another of the concerns shared by the fourth year students. So too is the direction of their effort. (On 'level and direction of effort', cf. Becker *et al.* 1961.) In other words they are preoccupied with the amount of work and effort demanded from them, and the sort of tasks at which they are required to work. (This sort of concern was also one of the most, if not the single most, pressing of the topics dealt with by the student culture at the Kansas medical school.) As one might expect, the various cliniques, by virtue of their different approaches to medicine or surgery, and their different commitments to teaching, are seen to demand varying degrees of effort on the students' part.

It is by no means the case, however, that students seek out, or appreciate those clinical firms which are thought to have low expectations of their students or low levels of productivity. On the contrary, those units which are identified as 'lazy' in their approach are avoided if possible for that very reason. Some students in fact appear to be almost masochistic in this respect - expecting to be worked hard on their clinical attachments and annoyed if they are not. As I have indicated already, the first year of clinical study is seen as less gruelling than the traumatic preparation for the '2nd MB' at the end of the previous year. And the students are grateful for that, but they certainly do not value too easy a ride.

This perspective derives from a rational calculation (and of course has nothing to do with masochism really). They recognise that the experience gained in the fourth year will be a most important grounding in the basics of clinical work. They are therefore justifiably concerned that, given the apparent variability of cliniques, they should find themselves attached to units which prepare them adequately and expose them to the necessary range of experience in sufficient depth. This has a bearing on their training and on their careers in general. The fourth year is the time when they should be laying the foundations of sound technique, basic knowledge and so on. They are also concerned with shorter term issues: they need to make sure that they are adequately prepared and 'covered' for the clinical examinations at the end of the year. One atrocity story which was circulating at the time of the fieldwork was related about a certain surgical unit. It was claimed that all those who had been attached to the unit had failed the relevant examination. It was clearly to be avoided on those grounds, students advised each other to steer clear of it, and it was held up as a dreadful warning against a careless choice of clinique. (During the fieldwork itself there was no evidence of such a correlation between specific attachments and examination failures: but these myths defy such sober facts.)

In fact it is not at all easy for students to evaluate whether they have achieved the appropriate experience and mastery. There is no precisely defined syllabus for the clinical instruction. There are broad aims which are clearly recognised: the development of competence in the basic skills such as history-taking and physical examination, and an ability to recognise the signs or symptoms of a variety of diseases. But there is no specific indication of what fourth year students should have done, should have witnessed, or should know about. Consequently, their evaluation of their progress must take place in something of a vacuum. A constant comparison of one's own range of experience against that of other students is therefore of considerable importance.

The fact that the curriculum of clinical instruction remains to a considerable extent unwritten and implicit is in large measure a direct reflection of the basic character of such clinical work. It must depend very largely on the routine practice of the units concerned, the availability of patients with relevant disorders and so on. In the nature of things, the exact nature and timing of clinical work is unpredictable and it would not normally be possible for it to be specified in detail in advance. Clinicians cannot readily legislate for the presence and sequence of patients who may come under their care. The actual content of a student's experience on any individual clinique, and hence over the entire year, is uncertain. All the information that students have to go on in planning an undergraduate career, and in evaluating their progress rests on the shared stock of knowledge and experience enshrined in the student culture.

The foregoing considerations do not mean that all students go flat out to attend units which demand the very highest effort. For the most part they seek to balance the level of effort. Some individuals clinicians, or their firms, are felt to be *too* demanding.

As I have emphasised, the first days on the wards constitute a major transition in the students' careers: while welcomed, it is an experience which brings its own demands. The novelty of the setting, the acquisition of new skills, the exposure to patients, are all felt to be potentially stressful. The first contacts with patients can seem, by turn, exciting, traumatic, enjoyable or depressing. Hence many of the students appreciate what they describe as a 'fairly gentle' introduction to this uncharted territory, in an atmosphere which is not too taxing on their intellectual and emotional resources. Cliniques are valued in so far as they provide a 'relaxed' atmosphere for the introduction to clinical studies.

Cliniques which are not relaxed are described as 'high powered'. In terms of students' typifications, the 'central' cliniques in the Royal Infirmary are felt to be more 'high powered' than those in the 'periphery' (a view which is in keeping with the other perceptions of clinique atmosphere already outlined). The staff at The Royal are believed to expect more of their students, in terms of the amount of new material they are required to assimilate, the pace of the teaching, and the amount of formal instruction provided. (In fact there is rather more time available for teaching at the Royal Infirmary than elsewhere: some time is lost in transporting the students to peripheral hospitals.) The typical sort of comment offered about the experience of the Royal is that students there are 'thrown in at the deep end' of clinical work. Units elsewhere are described as providing a more gradual start. For example:

> Over coffee it came out that the students had gathered there are differences between the [peripheral] Hospital and the Royal Infirmary. They told me that they were being introduced to clinical experience 'fairly gently', whilst those at the Infirmary were being 'pushed in at the deep end'.

Over and above the fact that the majority of them are central, the professorial units are said to be particularly high powered. This is in accordance with their perceived academic orientation. Professorial units are thought of as being especially demanding, and to exercise exceptionally strong control over the students' work. Their distinctive atmosphere is sometimes spoken of as 'hothouse'. For this reason, some students try to avoid units of this sort. The hothouse atmosphere is related to the competitiveness which students believe characterises such academic settings: in the face of such (supposed) competition and rivalry, the staff members' demeanour is held to imply a display of superior academic fire-power, as the clinicians vie for kudos.

The students are also keen to gain *general* experience, rather than being exposed to an overspecialised and restricted range of clinical matters. In broad terms all the firms which students attend are general, but 'some are more general than others'. Students sometimes grumble that their introduction to clinical medicine or surgery is unbalanced because their clinical teachers spend too much time on their specialised work. On one surgical unit, for instance, students grumbled that they knew 'all there is to know about colostomies', but had not covered other aspects of more general interest. In this context too the students are interested in a close evaluation of the quality of educational experience which they acquire in the course of their attachment to various clinical firms in the teaching hospitals.

Cliniques and careers

In addition to the need for the immediate choice of fourth year units, there may be significant considerations to be kept in mind concerning future contingencies. This arises from the element of patronage in the organisation of medical careers (cf. Hall, 1948), which is of crucial relevance towards the end of the students' undergraduate course, when they must seek posts as house-physicians and house-surgeons during their pre-registration year.

The particular hospitals and clinical firms where a student undertakes this year of work can be of considerable importance in the development of his or her subsequent career and attainment within medicine. To complete a house job successfully in a teaching hospital which enjoys high prestige is an important first step on the ladder of a successful career in the medical profession. Similarly, to be employed in the firm of a well known and important consultant is an important career contingency.

For a student with any degree of ambition, then, the prospect of obtaining a favourable house job in one of the popular firms in an Edinburgh teaching hospital is a consideration to be borne in mind. It may be seen as an important goal to be attained at the end of the student's undergraduate career. Not all the fourth-year students actively consider their pre-registration year, but of those who do the majority believe that it is desirable to complete at least one of the house jobs in one of Edinburgh's hospitals. To leave and go elsewhere might look less well in the future: it might suggest that one has not been considered good enough to be offered a post by any of the clinicians who have a close personal knowledge of one's work as a student. One of the male students I talked to articulated this concern, and I summarised our conversation in my field notes:

> For his pre-registration year he would probably stay in Edinburgh, and at the moment the [peripheral] hospital was an appealing proposition. Staying in Edinburgh was important, otherwise, when one is applying for jobs,

people would ask you why you didn't do a house job in your teaching area. On the whole he thought this was unfortunate, as he would like to move about more freely. He said that when consultants are looking for housemen to look after their patients they will naturally prefer the student they know; they will therefore be most likely to take someone who has worked under them for a final year attachment. He added, 'maybe it's just an old boy tradition'. He repeated that one's final year attachments are important for where you do your house job. Some people, he told me, even get their house-jobs fixed very early, even immediately after their summer clerkships. He also told me that there is more care taken over Final Phase attachments than in choosing junior cliniques.

The selection of successful candidates for house jobs, as the students see it, depends very largely on their personal relationships with the consultant staff of their Final Phase units. The jobs are seen as being largely in the hands of the chief of the firm, and the successful application for a job could depend on a student's being 'well in' with the clinicians concerned.

Future success in medicine is therefore seen to depend largely on creating a good impression with a consultant under whom one would like to train during one's first postgraduate year, and perhaps subsequently, should one become a senior house officer, registrar and so on. In other words, the most advantageous transition to postgraduate teaching is seen by the students as being a process of sponsored mobility. In order to maximise one's chances of such sponsorship and recruitment, it may be necessary to manage one's self-presentation with some care (cf. Goffman, 1971). Impression management on the part of the students can therefore be geared towards creating a favourable impression with staff members, as prospective sponsors and professional superiors. For instance, after a conversation with two students (one male, one female) I noted:

They both agreed that getting on in a specialty depended on what one of them called 'the coefficient between ability and getting on with the clinical staff'. You can, one of them said, be a surgeon of moderate ability and yet be successful because 'you happen to click with a surgeon', or you can be a very good surgeon and fail to get on because of poor relations with members of staff.

These students were expecting this 'coefficient' to be of importance in their later experiences in the medical school, and in their subsequent careers, should they find themselves committed to a career in a hospital speciality. Another male student I interviewed was similarly explicit about the process, although he wished to disassociate himself from the practice of impression management:

> St.   People feel it's time to impress people. There's a
>   lot of this goes on, I don't really like it.
> P.A.   What do people do?
> St.   The occasional 'sir', being nice, not being
>   obstreperous, being benign and harmless.

He added that he suspected that a lot of clinicians could 'see through' this sort of impression management on the students' part, so that it was not always totally effective. He also stressed that it was not really an effective strategy at the fourth year stage, being more relevant for the students in their final year.

> St.   You try to pick a final year attachment where you
>   want to do a house job, and then you turn on the
>   charm.

Just as this student sought to distance himself from these practices, so do many of his peers. An awareness of this career strategy is admitted to by many students, but it is something that is generally attributed to others; it is 'something that goes on' rather than 'something we do'. Students are reticent about appearing over keen or 'pushy' in the eyes of the fellow members of the clinique. During the fourth year, competition for attention and recognition is not pressing. To push oneself forward at this stage may be to risk contravention of the students' collective levels and directions of effort. But, as the following extract from my field notes suggests, this consideration may be oriented to by students in their interaction with clinicians:

> The group were discussing whether or not they were going
> to go and hear their chief, who was giving that week's
> clinical lecture for the final hour that morning. Roy
> Bateson was in a bad mood and seemed genuinely
> unwilling to go along. One of his fellow students said he
> reckoned that it all depended on whether he wanted to

'keep in' with Dr. Crosbie, with an eye to his future career.

The implication of this was that the student's absence from the lecture might well be noted by the chief, and might be remembered and held against him subsequently. This group of students were in fact approaching the matter in a fairly lighthearted way. Nevertheless, they did appear to be voicing a genuine concern over career management.

One student in particular drew attention to the importance of the informal criteria which students may have to bear in mind in thinking about their careers, and their implications for practice beyond qualification. Our conversation had turned to why people opt for an 'honour year':

> St. I think the major reason people go into them is that they realise that it'll help them get a job later.
>
> P.A. Is that true?
>
> St. Well I think, I mean, we're all churned out at the same level: you know there's no classes in the MB ChB, so I think if you've got other things that you can hold out, like honours Pathology or something, it'll help you get a good post. There's a lot of other ways of doing it, though. One of the most recent ones I've heard of in the final year if you do a locum, a week or so, it gets you well known and well liked. That's when you do it well of course; if you kill a patient they're not going to be too happy.

As this student describes so well, there is a recurrent problem facing the career conscious student. As one of a large number of students he or she can feel relatively anonymous. Few can reasonably expect to be outstanding academically and to impress members of staff on their examination performances alone. Yet the allocation of first hospital posts is often felt to depend upon the personal choice of the consultants on the various wards. As one student told me, 'It depends largely on how many people you impress' as to how successful a student is in his or her applications for house posts. As is apparent in the extracts I have already quoted, students do not deny the relevance of academic ability and qualifications (honours degrees and distinctions in examinations are recognised as depending upon intellectual ability). Rather, they suggest that in themselves they may not be sufficient conditions for success, however necessary. Ability must be matched by careful career management and some success in 'fronting' (cf. Olesen and Whittaker, 1968 p.173 ff.).

While these considerations filter down to students in the fourth year, the topic of house jobs impinges on their immediate plans in a rather indirect way. To be precise, it informs a strategy of *avoiding* certain units rather than seeking them out. The rationality for this procedure is derived from a simple rule: in the normal run of events, students are not admitted to units for their final year attachments if they have already been there for their fourth year teaching. In other words, attachment to a clinical unit for a fourth-year clinique will normally preclude attachment to that same unit in the student's last year. The students' strategies of clinique choice are (or may be) formulated with this in mind.

There may, therefore, be some conflict in students' decision making. They need to reconcile the dilemma of opting directly for popular and attractive units, and deliberately avoiding them in the hope of being able to obtain an attachment in one or more of them in their final year (when the pay-off may be of greater and more lasting significance). A strongly fancied unit may not be put down as a preference, but may be 'saved up' for the later part of the undergraduate course. During the closing weeks of my second term's observation, for instance, I noted students employing this tactic in coming to decisions about clinique choices for the coming term:

> I overheard a fifth year girl giving another girl advice about possible attachments to try for in her term of surgery. She named two of these possible cliniques, but added that her friend should do her best to keep one of them back for her final year attachment.

Similarly, in discussing how she had chosen her first medical unit, one of the female students told me that in doing so, she had 'done a bit of asking around' with students in the year above her. They had told her that the unit she picked would offer her 'a good start' in clinical medicine.

This aspect of clinique choice was also displayed by other students during the year:

> Gerald Kennedy had deliberately steered clear of [peripheral] Hospital, so that for his final year his chances are good for getting an attachment there. He explained that you have to do eight weeks in the Royal Infirmary anyway,

so it is a good idea to keep options open for the peripheral units. His general planning is to be in the [peripheral] Hospital, as he would like to get a house job there. The____Hospital is 'no good to anybody', and as for the__ Hospital, 'you have to be a certain type, beer swilling and back slapping'.

One of the female students I interviewed also articulated this concern:

P.A.   How did you pick [her present unit]?
St.   It was mainly ... going on previous reports. The fact that I didn't want to come to the Royal until the last term, but I didn't want to come to the [peripheral] again, 'cos I wanted to leave various options open for the final year. It's all a question of fiddling things, isn't it?

If students should fail to obtain an attachment to the units of their preference in the first clinical year, or if they discover that a chosen unit does not suit them, or is not all its reputation led them to expect, then the perspective of 'deferred gratification' can be turned to good account. While present experience may be judged unsatisfactory, students can reconcile themselves to this by the thought that at least it is now 'out of the way'. The rule against returning to a fourth year unit can therefore be seen as protecting the student against having to repeat the experience. This can be illustrated from my field notes. During a coffee-time conversation between two final year students and a few fourth years, I heard them talking about this aspect of student careers. They had just been taught by the chief of their firm, who had been particularly severe and critical with one of the older students:

A senior, who had been rather picked on by Dr. Burton, said he thought he had been like that because he hadn't wanted Dr. Burton's house job. The conversation turned to house jobs in general. One of the seniors told the fourth-years that one wants to end up in The Royal for one's final year attachment (as they had done). The two seniors were in agreement that the fourth year students were lucky in having got Dr. Burton's attachment 'out of the way' early in the course. John Cartwright (one of the fourth years) told them that Dr. Burton's firm had been his third choice for medicine, and he had wanted to do surgery this term anyway.

In such a fashion, apparently unlucky students in the fourth year can 'cool out' their own apparent lack of success. The otherwise poor start of finding oneself on an unpopular clinique can be reinterpreted as a fortunate contingency, as an instance of luck rather than the reverse. In this way the appearance of a favourable and rational career pattern can be salvaged and reassembled by the employment of a deferred gratification perspective on cliniques and clinique choices.

Counting experience

I have described how students attempt to plan their undergraduate careers, in order to optimise the experience they gain of clinical work. I have also described how they evaluate the experience they and their fellow students actually gain. Since there is no set guide to precisely what they should encounter, then the students have to engage in a form of research in order to gauge the range of variation. Only in this way can they place their own individual experience in context. The research strategy they use, and it is one which is familiar to sociologists, is that of the 'constant comparative method'. On the basis of their folk model of the teaching hospitals, the students compare surgical and medical, central and peripheral, professorial and non-professorial cliniques.

I have outlined some of these student comparisons above, and I have detailed some of them elsewhere (Atkinson, 1973 and 1974). Here I am less concerned with the actual detailed comparisons between hospitals and specialties than with the more general implications of this continuous assessment which fourth-year students, individually and collectively, produce. What they are doing is 'counting clinical experience'. David Sudnow (1967), in his study of death in hospitals, provides us with a parallel, and indeed touches on medical education directly. In a discussion of how deaths on the ward are treated as newsworthy, reportable events, Sudnow remarks:

New student nurses and, apparently, young medical students make it a habit of counting such events as deaths, and locate their own growing experience and sophistication by reference to 'how many times' such and such has been encountered, witnessed, done, etc. Throughout the medical

> world, numerical representations of phenomena are
> accorded central status as marks of experience. (p.37)

Sudnow goes on to note that there comes a point in one's sophistication when individual events are no longer counted, when one begins to 'lose count'.

The fourth year medical students, being novices still, are mostly at the stage of 'counting' their clinical experiences. Specific events, and more general features (such as clinique 'atmosphere') are all added to the store of experience. There is, as I have said, no pre-given corpus of knowledge and experience which the students have to 'put under their belt'. Insofar as they recognise and assemble such a corpus, they have to 'make it up as they go along'. They do, however, come to know that there are many things that they might reasonably learn to do, see done, or at least learn about.

It is a source of great satisfaction to students when they acquire a new experience. The train-spotter offers one analogy here; another is the stereotypical tourist, who 'does' the approved sights (MacCannell, 1977). There was, for instance, one student who was in residence at one of the hospitals as a living-in clerk (an opportunity available to a few junior students). His duties as a clerk included the collection of blood samples early each morning. He lost no opportunity to drop into conversation references to 'when I was taking bloods this morning', and to draw attention to the fact that his fellow students did not share the opportunity for such 'real' clinical experience. On one occasion I came across another student who was quite made up as a result of mistaken identity. A junior doctor had mistaken him for a more senior student, and had asked him to carry out a simple test on one of the patients. He had been asked to examine a patient's stool for traces of faecal occult blood. The student had not 'let on' that he has only a fourth-year, and he was clearly very pleased at this opportunity. Ward tasks of this sort are, of course, menial. They are not the sort of thing which the students will continue to carry out eagerly. Indeed they will probably be all too pleased to delegate them to future cohorts of junior students themselves. The students at Kansas (Becker *et al.*, 1961, p.259) complained at being given such 'scut work' to carry out. The novice students at Edinburgh only 'count' such experiences at the very outset of their clinical work. Early experiences are stored up and they are treasured to begin with. As time goes by, so students start to differentiate their experiences with greater discrimination. Of course, the collection and narration of personal experience are not confined to the emergent careers of students and young doctors. The rehearsal of personal experience is a stock-in-trade of the senior clinician too. The expression of personal reminiscence, personal preference and personal experience is a recurrent theme in clinical discourse and clinical instruction. In counting and treasuring their clinical experiences, the junior medical students are no different from their more senior professional mentors and colleagues. Their acquisition of a biographically-grounded stock of clinical experience is a significant aspect of their socialisation.

There are many clinical procedures which the students are eager to witness. These include: lumbar punctures; putting up a drip; taking samples of bone marrow; taking blood pressure; passing catheters. Their eagerness to witness clinical tasks is most pressing on surgery cliniques. If possible they are usually keen to be shown how to do such things, and to practise at least some of them themselves. Such achievements are all counted and recounted to others. In themselves, many of these valued experiences are routine work for others, and are the sort of thing which these selfsame students will soon 'lose count of'. By the time they qualify such experiences will have become mundane for them, as they are for all competent and experienced practitioners. For the time being, however, the students are frustrated and have few opportunities to witness or to try routine clinical tasks. Their teachers insist on treating these practical accomplishments and spectacles as unduly trivial to be included in the teaching for these junior students. The acts themselves are so thoroughly taken-for-granted that clinicians never think to explain them or have them demonstrated. The students, on the other hand, are greedy for experience, and are sometimes afraid that they may find themselves at some future time with major gaps in their basic clinical grounding.

On occasion, enterprising students use their own initiative to search out extra experience. For instance, one or two make it their business to get to know casualty officers and to visit the Accident and Emergency department in their own time. Here they see front-line medicine, much as they do on waiting nights, of a sort very different from what they see during normal bedside teaching. There the students may get the chance to clean, dress and stitch wounds. They are allowed to learn and practise on simple enough injuries, and the casualty officers are no doubt glad enough to get their voluntary help.

As I have described already, in addition to these specific clinical experiences, the students evaluate their cliniques in terms of general atmosphere. Crucial to such evaluations is the degree to which the students are made to feel incorporated into the clinical firm, and establish satisfying working relationships with doctors and patients. There has been a debate in the literature on the status of the medical student - whether he or she is to be portrayed as a 'junior colleague', or a 'boy (or girl) in white'. What the Edinburgh students experience is that they enjoy no single status. Sometimes they are treated as junior partners, at other times their passive, marginal position is stressed: Shuval (1975) makes this point in relation to her research in Israel.

What is important to the fourth-year students is the extent to which they can feel part of what is going on on the wards, and can feel that they are, medically speaking, where the action is. Their participation in the reality of the hospital wards and clinics is the touchstone by the which their educational and clinical experience is judged. The clinical phase of study is eagerly welcomed on this basis. Although students' ideals are not lived up to equally on all units, their first year of clinical work is, as we have seen, a major turning point. The appeal of the clinical lies in its apparent authenticity, and its rationale in the students' exposure to medical reality.

5 The clinical setting

Clinical teaching on the hospital wards derives from an apprenticeship mode of professional socialisation. Although medical students are not working employees in the organisation, they are taught in the work milieu, in the 'real world' of medicine. To some extent, as they process round the wards with a teacher, or work individually whilst clerking patients, the students are involved in the day to day world of medical work. Yet at the same time they are not unequivocally members of the ward personnel and participants in their routine work. It is not so much that they are incompetent recruits, but rather that the students do not have responsibility for any aspect of the patient's daily care. Their position in the hospital is therefore ambiguous. The teaching encounter at a patient's bedside is to some degree defined as a medical one: in some ways the work of the teacher and the students is kept distinct from the rest of the ward and its routine; to some extent therapeutic and educational work are in competition with each other. This chapter will explore these facets of the clinical teaching encounter.

The medical milieu and ambience must be accomplished and sustained as a prerequisite to the specifically educational tasks at the bedside. The production of a medical encounter will therefore be considered first. As Emerson (1970) has pointed out, 'situations differ in how much effort it takes to sustain the current definition of the situation', and she cites the gynaecological examination as one which is extremely precarious. I believe that she attributes specifically to gynaecological examinations many features that are common to most, if not all, medical encounters. Certain aspects of medical work require a degree of careful reality management on the part of medical personnel - and this applies whether the situation is a 'delicate' internal examination or a 'straightforward' out-patient visit, or indeed a session with medical students. Emerson comments on a number of reality sustaining (or creating) devices in her discussion of gynaecologists and their patients. She points to the fact that

93

the medical definition is expressed by a number of indicators: that the interaction is located in a medical milieu, the hospital clinic or doctor's office, for instance. Within that space, decor and equipment complete the medical *mise en scene*: 'The staff wear medical uniforms, don medical gloves, use medical instruments'. Similarly, the presence of medical personnel and the exclusion of lay members 'helps to preclude confusion between the contact of medicine and the contact of intimacy'.

Emerson also discusses the use of linguistic conventions in sustaining a medical definition of the situation - for instance, the substitution of the definite article for pronominal adjective ('the vagina', not 'your vagina'), or 'delicate' periphasis ('down below' to refer to the pelvic region, etc.). Along with a degree of impersonality, Emerson also points out, the examining doctor must attempt to produce a demeanour suggesting care and concern. She goes on to describe a number of ways in which such a smooth accomplishment of the examination may be threatened, and how such threats may be neutralised by physicians, nurses, or other personnel.

I have dwelt at some length on Emerson's description of the gynaecological examination and its routine accomplishment in order to make the following point: *mutatis mutandis*, Emerson's description applies equally to most, if not all, medical encounters - and certainly those that take place in a medical locale. In all such encounters the medical ambience hedges round the actors' construction of reality; in all cases the medical personnel are there, often with other professionals and auxiliary workers at hand; in all cases the talk and demeanour of the professionals sustains the medical reality. What I am arguing is that Emerson's paper in fact presents a generalised picture of medical reality in a professionalised setting, and I take it as a general introduction to the construction of medical reality.

This was brought home to me in the context of what was in fact a delicate, personal examination rather like Emerson's gynaecological encounter. It occurred in the course of a surgery ward round. We were at the bedside of a man in his thirties who had a swollen and painful testicle. After presenting the case briefly, the consultant asked one of the female students to examine the patient's swollen scrotum. I observed very few bedside teaching sessions in which such examinations of patients' genitals had been involved: I was therefore particularly on the alert for the sort of things described by Emerson, such as methods of guarding against embarrassment, or repair work when embarrassment occurs. The examination I was observing was delicate in two senses, as it involved a young woman examining a man's genitals, and it was, potentially, extremely painful for the patient and called for careful examination by the student. Immediately after the teaching session I noted:

> I wondered if she would show any embarrassment at examining the patient's genitals. She blushed a little, but I could detect no other signs of embarrassment on her part.

I was not able to observe any signs of particular embarrassment, or of affected nonchalance and matter of factness on the part of the patient:

> Observation, concerning Joan Emerson. She discusses the 'clinical' approach as minimising embarrassment. But such an approach happens anyway - i.e. in all cases, not only in those which involved sexual encounters which might be open to misinterpretation. In other words, students will generally adopt a 'serious' and 'considerate' approach to the patient. It would be difficult to imagine what behavioural differences one could expect from situations of heightened 'threat' or 'embarrassment' ....

At this point in my observations, then, I was drawing attention to the fact that Emerson's comments are not confined to gynaecology in their relevance to medical encounters. Rather, they should be seen as describing a special case, throwing into relief features which are general to all doctor-patient interactions. In Emerson's terms, the gynaecologist's talk and demeanour can be seen as informing the patient, 'Look, this is perfectly ordinary clinical encounter - a perfectly normal and routine examination'. But the very fact that it comes over as normal and routine depends upon the fact that this is the nature of all (or most) run-of-the-mill clinical encounters.

The construction of bedside teaching is a variant of medical reality management, and we can see how many of the devices that Emerson identifies are mobilised or are available. The medical ambience does not need construction as a background feature. It is already constituted in the hospital, and patients will already have been socialised into the medical situation by the time they are visited by the clinician and his students. They will at least have been admitted and examined by the resident physician and will have been worked on by the nursing staff. In the same way, there is no need for the explicit recruitment of medical or auxiliary staff to create a medical definition: they are routinely on hand - the house officers performing their day to day duties, the nurses and auxiliary staff theirs.

As part of this process, the medical student's uniform is an important dramaturgical prop. Putting on their white coat is an important symbolic manifestation of students' status passage from preclinical to clinical studies (cf. Becker *et al.*, 1961, p.194). Not only does it symbolise this new status to fellow students, it also declares the wearer of the white coat as a medical person to others in the hospital. For instance, it marks one off from such transients as visitors and out-patients, as one strides through the corridors from ward to ward. The white coat may ensure the wearer privileged access in the hospital; it is a passport as one moves about the building.

As a white-coated person myself, I was aware of the relative immunity it offered. It provided excellent camouflage as I wandered about, looking for students or their teachers. Indeed, on one occasion, I was rather disconcerted to find that my camouflage had worked too well. Whilst standing with a group of students, waiting for a doctor to teach, I was alarmed to find a member of the public tugging at my sleeve, telling me that a woman had just collapsed nearby, and asking for my help. Luckily I was able to get enthusiastic support from my knot of students; some went for help, whilst others rushed off eagerly to see and join in some real emergency medicine. For the students, too, the white coat confers medical status, and proclaims them as legitimate personnel to the patients and hospital staff. Along with the coat, the student's clinical instruments complete the picture of the young doctor.

The stethoscope, while having obvious pragmatic value, it also of great dramaturgical value in proclaiming the clinical student's new found place in the medical hierarchy. During the earliest days in the field, I noticed how stethoscopes were a topic of conversation. Several students pointed out to me how they and their colleagues displayed their stethoscope as a badge of office. Stethoscopes are carried in the roomy pockets of the white coat. But, my informants told me, the more junior students kept theirs clearly visible, left dangling artfully over the edge of the pocket, whereas more senior students would stuff their stethoscope further into their pockets, even out of sight. This, it was suggested to me, may imply that whereas the 'green' fourth-year students are eager for clinical work and involvement, their more world-weary seniors are as concerned to avoid them. Be that as it may, the stethoscope, plus the tendon hammer, are obvious emblems of the student's medical status. By the same token, their possession may reassure the novices and bolster their confidence in the strange new milieu of the hospital. For instance:

When we got to the hospital we went to the lockers. The students were laughing and joking, rather self consciously, I thought, about carrying stethoscopes. One said it was because he was hoping to use it soon, and added that it also boosted his confidence to be seen carrying it.

To go with their medical uniforms and trappings, further aspects of the students' self-presentation are related to his or her appearance as a medical person. To some extent, on entering the clinical years, students are expected to 'smarten themselves up'. During the preclinical years, the students of the medical school dress much like any other students. When they go on the wards, some 'standards' may be imposed.

One senior registrar mentioned to me that he sometimes 'looked twice' at students, and thought that if he were a patient, he would not fancy being treated by people who looked like that; he had never actually come across 'standards' that are normally required throughout all clinical units, however. These were outlined for some students I was with at an introductory meeting on the first morning in the hospital:

Dr Lukes went on to say that some of the students would have already visited the wards on a Saturday morning. He added that for their work on the wards the men were required to wear ties, although suits were not obligatory. Although, he explained, the doctors did not insist that men have their hair short, he suggested that men with long hair should tuck it into the collar of their white coat.

Similarly, in an introductory lecture one physician told the students that although 'faculty don't care', the patients 'tend to get upset if people are dressed in a peculiar way or have their hair down to here. They are to be comforted, not confronted'. It is noticeable that women's appearance was not specified. The only time when a female student's personal appearance was commented on occurred while the student were practising percussing the chest, in the first term on the wards. The young woman in question had long, carefully manicured nails, which were preventing her percussing properly with the finger tips. The consultant suggested that she should trim the nails, and I noted that she had done so by the following morning. Some of the female students appeared in trousers, and this was never adversely commented on.

There was in fact a wide range of personal styles and modes of dress current among the students, but observation across the years did suggest that as they progress through the medical school, they do tend to adopt a more sober and conventional apperance, even smarter clothes and hair styles. This was something which students themselves would sometimes point out to me, as they directed my attention to their more senior colleagues in and around the hospitals and the medical quadrangle. Although there was no miraculous overnight transformation, I did notice how students began to adopt the style of their senior colleagues. Particularly during the early days in the field I noticed that the male students would comment on and chaff each other about their clothes and hair styles. Thus, on the first morning of my first year's work, I noted the following interaction in the lecture theatre:

> One student entered in what was clearly a new jacket and tie; his hair was fairly long, but well trimmed. He went up to sit beside a friend who had shoulder length hair. Seizing it, he said, 'This lot will have to come off'. He then turned and pirouetted to show off his own new clothes.

In terms of the students' personal front (Goffman, 1971) this is part of their transformation from lay persons to medical professionals. In parallel with the doctrinal conversions (Davis, 1968) that student professionals go through, they must come to take on the manners (in the broadest sense) of the members of the occupational group. Transformations in self-perception are accompanied by transformations in the self that the students present to others about them - fellow students, teachers, and the patients on the wards. At the same time, we can see how this development relates directly to the bedside teaching, insofar as these students' impression management contributes to the successful definition of the situation as a legitimate medical one.

It is not only the students' appearance which is involved here. More generally, their *demeanour*, and that of the doctors involved, is an important constituent feature of the clinical teaching encounter. 'The bedside manner' is a general, common or garden way of expressing the range of behaviours that are typically expected as distinctive of medical practitioners. While such things are notoriously hard to pin down and document, their general effect is apparent as a background feature of bedside interactions.

Teachers coach students in several aspects of behaviour which are part of the normal demeanour of clinical medicine. An example of this is the injunction that the bed should be approached from the patient's right hand side. The *reason* for this piece of etiquette is never articulated, but it is often stated as a basic principle of bedside work. Although the requirement may be grounded in practical considerations, it is presented to the students more in the guise of a ceremonial act, rather than one based on convenience or comfort. Sitting on the patient's bed is also a breach of etiquette. It is permissible to perch on it to examine the patient's back; any 'sloppy' sitting on the bed lays a student open to reproof from a clinician.

In much the same vein is the injunction that students should get on the same level as the patient, although here the comfort of the patient is more clearly at issue; students should avoid towering over the patient. Similarly, students are told to make sure that their hands are not too cold when they palpate a patient's body. This can cause further problems, however. On one occasion a student, asked to examine a patient's abdomen, began to rub his hands together, to warm them up. The consultant told him, rather sharply, not to do that: 'It looks as if you're just about to sit down to a good dinner!' Students are also reminded to remake the bed if they have to pull the bedclothes off. This demonstrates consideration for both the patient and the nursing staff.

The observance of such etiquette is one way in which students are coached to respect and reproduce the appearances of medical work. More generally, however, the medical definition of reality requires that some rules of everyday interaction are set aside, and more context specific rules employed. The example of the gynaecological examination, referred to above, is a special case of the demands of such reality maintenance. Clinical work requires that patients' bodies be peered at, probed and felt. Such privileged access is normally confined to intimates, and as Lief and Fox (1963) comment:

> The amounts and occasions of body contact are carefully regulated in all societies, and very much so in ours. Thus, the kind of access to the body of the patient that a physician in our society has is a uniquely privileged one. Even in the course of so called physical examination, the physician is permitted to handle the patient's body in ways otherwise permitted to special intimates, and in the case of procedures such as rectal and vaginal examinations in ways not even permitted to a sexual partner.

99

Junior students do not normally perform vaginal examinations, though rectals are sometimes done. However, they are routinely expected to perform other sorts of physical examination. Such encounters have to be handled with some care: the participants need to make it clear to one another that this is a medical situation, and not an intimate one. This problem is not entirely confined to the medical arena, but can occur whenever contexts require intimate physical contact (e.g. bodily search by security guards). In all cases the smooth performance of such encounters requires that the actors should treat these events in a matter of fact way. In such interactions - including those involving the medical students - decorum calls for a posture of personal detachment coupled with a display of concern.

For the students, the successful accomplishment of bedside encounters requires that they learn two basic things. First, they must manage to treat the occasion as a 'normal', 'medical' one; secondly, they must maintain their composure in a semi-public display of their embryonic medical skills. For in their 'on the job' acquisition of competence in bedside work, the students usually have an audience. Inescapably, the patient, if conscious, is in a position to observe their efforts. Frequently, they have to perform with a clinician and their fellow students as an audience as well.

Students frequently encounter difficulties in composure when they first encounter patients on the wards. One student put it quite forcibly:

> It's a terrible experience, sort of interviewing patients for the first time ....

Other students put it rather less dramatically:

> I've never had any trouble with patients personally ... I think I can get on fairly well with most patients. I don't think anybody's ever complained about me .... I was very apprehensive. It's a bit worrying as a student to ask people questions about their personal life and private life, and go into personal problems. You're not qualified and they know you're not qualified. Very embarrassing to start with.
>
> You have to learn to conquer your initial shyness. That's the thing I found most difficult, because you feel that the patient expects so much of you. You know, because, in

their eyes, you're a doctor. And I felt that the first few sessions I was there I felt it acutely - that they were very embarrassed for me because I was obviously incompetent. And that was very difficult at first - and that was one of the first things we learnt: put on a calm front even though you haven't a *clue* what you're doing. The other thing is to express yourself ....

The same female student went on to say,

> I don't find it difficult on my own at all: that passed off pretty quickly. But I still find it difficult to interview a patient in front of the class. And this is very difficult, especially if you happen to be landed with a difficult patient .... I really came across my first difficult patient in front of the class .... I asked what was the matter and she, you know, she came back with the classic reply, 'You should know doctor'. And I was completely unprepared for it.

While students can manage to overcome their apprehensions over interviewing and examining patients, they find their performances before doctors and their fellow students more nerve racking. As one student said:

> At the ward meetings at the end of the week, they accepted you as part of the staff. And if you had a patient that was of interest, you had to present it to the ward, which was a frightening experience ....

And another of the students said,

> I don't mind at all having one patient, one person, but I don't like having surgeons breathing down your neck going 'Tut'.

The presence of clinicians therefore confronts the novice student with a critical audience for their incompetent first trials at clinical work.

While patients can also be a source of embarrassment to the students, they may appear to be more indulgent, and students' avowal of their novitiate status can be employed as a resource. During the early days of

101

students' time on the wards, they sometimes get lost in their question and answer sequences, and are forced to consult the small handbook provided by the medical school.

> Dr. Saunders said that I could go off with the students if I liked, and I trotted into the ward, where I found Denis Elliott interviewing a middle-aged man. Denis was referring to his little booklet on 'how to take a history', and he referred to it several times: as he did so he apologised to the patient for having to use it.

On such occasions students would offer rather nervous apologies for having to use this crib, whilst patients would acknowledge that they did not mind 'helping' the students. On other occasions, rather more 'covering up' can be employed by the students as they strive to find their bearings. As one of the students explained it to me:

> You thought of all the questions to ask and then forgot what to ask them next. I would talk about the weather - filling in the questions as I started to remember them again.

The prospect of a nurse as an audience can also produce fears of being 'shown up' as incompetent in students as they begin their clinical work:

> We all met again by the noticeboard. Jeremy Davies and David Dean were discussing their respective patients. Jeremy had been examining his female patient, and David asked him if he had had a nurse present. Jeremy replied that he wasn't going to show off his incompetence in front of any nurse - he wanted to preserve his 'aura of competence'. He asked if a nurse was necessary as a chaperone. David thought it wasn't obligatory, but that regulations varied from place to place.

Students' inept performances are not always the subject for distress. On the contrary, the potential problems of their incompetence can be defused by laughter, and dissolve into general hilarity. For instance, one student described how humour can arise:

St.   It'll all come with practice anyway; in the summer when we start clerkships, probably within a week, we'll be so good - so used to doing it - that it'll only take a couple of hours. Whereas I can only do the central nervous system in a couple of hours now. Ever seen anybody doing that?

P.A.   [untruthfully] No.

St.   You have to try and work out the field of vision, so you hold their head down and get them to look straight into your eye and cover one eye - they have to cover one eye - and then you say 'Tell me when you see my finger', and you turn like that with your finger till they see it moving, and down there till they see it moving ... [he demonstrated the tangle that a student can get into] .... It's not unknown for the patient to burst out laughing, taking the piss out of the poor student. I think that happened to Loraine Beckett, you know her. Of course she giggles so much anyway. I think when they both got started, the examination ended. Poor Loraine.

The presence of patients as audiences of bedside teaching clearly constitutes something of a problem for the students in the early days of their clinical work.

Insulation from the rest of the ward

The scenic and ecological arrangement of bedside teaching emphasises the two features of clinical education. Insofar as the teaching is located in a hospital setting, in some respects it does share features of medical situations. But against that background, the educational situation is to some extent distinct from the medical milieu. As it progresses, the teaching round seems almost completely insulated from the other goings on in the ward. It is, in Goffman's terms, an ecological huddle and as it moves from bed to bed in the ward it remains enclosed by its symbolic membrane, to take another of Goffman's terms (Goffman, 1961a).

As the students cluster round the doctor and the patient's bed they produce an inward looking gathering, with the patient as the point of focus. The action is divorced from the rest of the ward that surrounds the group. Frequently the symbolic membrane round the group is given physical reality as the curtains are drawn round the bed, or screens brought round to preserve the privacy of the situation, and the doctor and students crowd round inside the screens. The space round a patient's bed is usually severely limited: a small territory which marks the limit on any privacy. The invasion by a doctor and a group of students (up to twelve in number, sometimes plus a sociologist) creates a tight scrum, with the patient in the middle. The patient is entirely enclosed within the group. This huddle is very rarely intruded upon by the comings and goings of other people about the ward and the invisible boundary round them is seldom broken. The students appear on the ward, but they are not *of* the ward; they have no clear identity or function within it. Hence there is little or no call for the students to interact with other medical or paramedical personnel.

The hierarchical nature of ward life is also demonstrated in the separation between the teaching session and the rest of the ward. The clinician's authority and power ensure routine ward work will not impinge on the teaching session. During one round I noted:

> at about this point, there was a bit of a commotion as some
> hospital staff were doing something or other and chattering
> rather loudly. Dr. McLellan called out sharply to them,
> asking them to be a bit quieter.

As we were inside the screening curtains, I could not see exactly what was going on beyond the pale. Whether or not the noise was produced by important clinical work or was idle 'chit chat' I had no way of knowing. But on an occasion which followed a couple of days later, it was clear that the disturbance was the outcome of necessary ward work.

> At the nearby bed, porters and nurses were trying to get a
> patient out of bed and onto a trolley: he was very heavily
> built, and appeared to be in a semi-conscious state. There
> was a bit of a commotion, as there were four of the nurses
> and a porter trying to do it. Dr. Essex stopped teaching for
> a moment, and raised his voice against the noise, 'Excuse
> me do you think you could modify your voices a little?'

The noise did die down, and the teaching was able to continue. No explicit reference was made to the patient and what was being done to him. To some extent, then, the situation parallels that special type described by Goffman (1971, p.33), in which 'the setting follows along with the performers'. Goffman instances royal processions, funeral corteges and the like, and the ward round is rather similar to these peripatetic gatherings. Goffman goes on to suggest that 'In the main, these exceptions seem to offer some kind of extra protection for performers who are, or who have momentarily become, highly sacred'. The degree of sacredness attached to the teaching round depends to a large extent on the rank of the clinician in charge. The consultant can generate an aura of inviolable sanctity and exclusiveness, whereas the more junior grades of staff are less able to produce and sustain such a definition. In almost all cases, however, the ward round remains set apart from the rest of the ward.

It is in the nature of the insulation of the students from the rest of the ward that there is little interaction between them and the nursing staff. Apart from the occasional informal encounter, I observed next to no student-nurse contact. This is in sharp contrast to popular images of student activities. It appears to be widely held stereotype that medical students' work regularly brings them into contact with the younger members of the nursing staff - to their pleasure - and with the senior nursing staff - to their chagrin and discomfort. This is, of course, part of the romantic myth of the general hospital, where nurses are attractive and sexually available to the male members of staff (cf. Atkinson, 1971), and which is fostered repeatedly in popular literature, film and television. It also reflects an earlier era when doctors and their students were predominantly male.

The students in their first clinical year have few working relationships with nurses and other hospital staff. The lack of contacts between students and nursing staff was also noted by Becker *et al.* (1961, p.197) in their study of Kansas. They also note that popular notions of medical training tend to overstress the importance of the nurses' role, and the rate of interaction between students and nurses, and they also suggest that the idea 'may possibly derive from the very much larger role she plays in the work lives of interns and residents'.

In the first instance, then, the teaching round is distinct from the routine work of the wards; it does not enter into the day to day therapeutic work being performed on the patient. The rounds and bedside lessons I observed were almost all *teaching* rounds, conducted by just one clinician with a group of students. This is in contrast with the traditional stereotype of the junior students tagging along behind the consultant and an entourage of registrars and housemen, ward sister and nurse, occasionally being thrown by a scrap of information as the consultant checks the progress of his patients. In contrast with this grandiose and flamboyant picture, the bedside teaching and ward rounds I observed were generally subdued affairs. The instruction of fourth year students was, usually, separated from clinicians' ward rounds. Very rarely did nurse or ward sister participate. On occasions when pressure of work or staffing shortages meant that teaching and routine ward work had to be conflated, or where the clinician designated to teach had to perform routine duties, this was taken as an untoward occurrence by the clinicians and an occasion for apologies. For instance:

> Today I went along at 11.15, as the students were doing
> individual ward work until that time. We then were due to be
> taught by Dr. Harvey: when he arrived he said that we would
> have to join his ward round, and he was afraid that the juniors
> would be getting 'a rather raw deal' out of it, and they should butt
> in and ask questions if there was anything they didn't understand.

The fact that I personally felt uncomfortable in this situation brought home to me the division between the everyday clinical round and the teaching session. Faced with the former I felt an intruder, in contrast to feeling relatively at home in the latter situation. The continuation of my field notes also underlines the non-teaching aspects of the round. Although Dr. Harvey, in apologising for the morning's arrangement, had asked the fourth year students to chip in with questions, I recorded after the round:

> In the fact there was relatively little questioning on the part
> of the students, and Dr. Harvey did not question them on
> many occasions.

I am not suggesting that there is necessarily no educational benefit in students' participation in such an exercise, simply that it is not treated as a scheduled part of the teaching programme.

On the other hand, I did record events connected with that ward round which were clearly to do with the day-to-day clinical work of the ward:

> One old lady had a haematological disorder which was
> puzzling the physicians. They had ordered a wide variety
> of tests to be carried out, and the time we spent at her
> bedside was mainly devoted to the consultant and the

106

junior doctors rifling through the case notes to try to sort out what had been done and what had been discovered.

Another old lady had been admitted with severe diarrhoea. The houseman wanted Dr. Harvey to see her particularly. I could hear the houseman tell Dr. Harvey that she had been seen on a previous occasion, but they had been unable to do anything. On Saturday she had been feeling very unwell, very depressed and very much sick and tired of doctors. The hospital had refused to admit her again and her GP had managed to get her admitted to the Royal Infirmary. Dr. Harvey looked very cross indeed and snapped, 'In other words, the GP has passed his problem on to us!'

Whilst this was going on, another houseman came up from the ward downstairs, and told Dr. Harvey that a patient had just died. He said something to the effect that their guesses were getting better, and that the patient had died more or less as and when expected. The houseman added that he thought that Dr. Jarvis would like to remove some of the organs: it was necessary to get them fresh, and they had to be taken in a couple of hours. Dr. Harvey said that if Dr. Jarvis would care to arrange that himself, that was alright, otherwise it could 'go through as normal'. The houseman said he would 'phone Dr. Jarvis, and would also get in touch with the Medical Superintendent for the permission of the next of kin.

Such features as these I have reported from my notes did not normally intrude upon the teaching scene. It was occasionally the case that clinical duties would compete with a doctor's teaching commitment, but it was more frequently resolved by the absence of the doctor (called away by his 'bleeper', for instance) rather than by a conflation of teaching and routine work.

The management of the intrusion of such work upon clinical teaching is also demonstrated by the following extract from my notes:

Dr. Raymond told me, slightly apologetically, that this wouldn't be a very formal session, as he would talk about some stuff they had been doing last week, and he now wanted the students to start thinking about the relative importance of the various methods of examining a patient's chest. Also, he said, he would be stopping to discuss something with Dr. Gill [the senior consultant].

He then took his group of students to the bedside of a patient in the male ward, and set them examining him. My notes continue:

> Whilst the students completed their examination, Dr. Raymond was talking to Dr. Gill and the other members of the chief's ward round. I could overhear some of their conversation, and could hear that Dr. Raymond was telling Dr. Gill about the same patient as he was teaching on. When he rejoined the group of students Dr. Raymond had a few words with me, telling me that he had to try to strike a balance between the needs of teaching and the management of his patients.

I observed something of the same sort in surgical units. On one occasion, for example, one of the surgeons was due to teach a small group I had attached myself to. When he came to find us, he explained rather apologetically that he had routine work to get on with, and this made his teaching difficult. The problem was that he needed to take blood from a patient and test the blood gases on a regular schedule of half hourly periods, which made it hard for him to give the students his full attention. In fact he took the students along with him while he performed the simple procedure and they watched while he did it. Between blood samples he talked to them about the patient and the test he was carrying out on her. As a matter of fact, the students seemed to be quite happy to observe the procedure and follow on while the surgeon went about his work. This was so to such an extent that when the clinician returned to the patient at the end of the teaching session, he clearly expected the students to leave him and wander off; but he was surprised to find them coming with him once more, to see the patient yet again. Although the doctor seemed to assume that the students would not appreciate this routine work, his assumption was not borne out. In the event there appeared to be no reason why he should have apologised to his students. Yet he did so, on the basis that they were not going to have a specially prepared and laid on teaching session. (Students in fact appreciate such opportunities to 'see things done'.) Such remedial exchanges (Goffman, 1972, pp. 124 ff.) highlight how some varieties of clinical education are normally segregated from the routine work of the hospital ward. This is particularly true of the bulk of bedside teaching: apologies and explanations appear to be appropriate if the two become confused.

The conduct of teaching in the course of ongoing medical work does occur in a number of relatively well defined contexts. These are primarily the operating theatre, out-patient departments and waiting nights. On such occasions the students are present whilst the doctor works on a patient as part of his normal medical work. Whereas the main preoccupation of the teaching rounds is educational, in these types of encounter the educational tasks must take second place to the diagnostic or therapeutic goals being pursued by the medical staff.

Yet even in these contexts, interaction between students and the hospital staff is minimised. In the out-patient clinic, for instance, the location of the consultation within the consulting room or cubicle means that the situation is one which remains confined to the clinician, students and patient. Again, it provides little or no opportunity for the students to engage in routine interaction with hospital personnel outside that focused group.

In the operating theatre the students also tend to be segregated. By and large they do not participate on the operating theatre floor, and do not therefore interact with the operating team members such as the theatre sister, the scrub nurse, anaesthetist and so on. Either in an open gallery or behind glass they may be spoken to by the operating surgeon, and may be called upon to answer questions on anatomy or surgical technique. But they take little or no active part in the proceedings on the theatre floor: they are observers of the action. But unlike the action that students observe and participate in on the teaching round, at least here the students can observe the real work of the surgical unit rather than specially contrived teaching situations.

Students are least segregated from the routine life of the ward when they attend on waiting nights. As I have already described, the students come into their respective clinical units during the late afternoon or during the evening and can stay well into the night. (How long they *do* stay depends on their personal interest and motivation, and the amount of action that is going on to hold them there: some nights can be very quiet, others very busy.) On these evenings, they are present when new patients are admitted with acute conditions. They therefore have more opportunity to see the work of junior hospital doctors as they admit the patients, take a history and perform a physical examination, and initiate any treatment that is appropriate. On occasion the students may themselves be allowed to take a patient's history. This opportunity to be 'where the action is' represents an important feature in students' perspective on their clinical instruction and experience.

The point that I have been making is that in some ways clinical teaching is kept distinct from the normal work of the hospital. This can be illustrated further by a consideration of the scheduling and timetabling of clinical work and bedside teaching. In the first place, a great deal of the work in the wards is *routine*. The daily round of the patient's life is marked by a recurrent cycle of management by the doctors, nurses and other staff. Although it does not fit Goffman's ideal type exactly, the general hospital displays some features of the total institution (Goffman, 1968). The hospital shares with other institutions of this type the fact that it is an all-encompassing organisation. For the inmates (the in patients, that is) the hospital as a complex organisation orders and regulates their life for twenty four hours a day. It is a relatively enclosed community; obviously, it is not so rigidly segregated as a monastery or prison (two varieties that Goffman uses to exemplify the notion) but for the patient in bed, the outside world is not directly accessible, and its representatives (his or her visitors) may only appear for limited periods and at set times. Again, from the patient's point of view, the hospital shares this similarity with the total institution: the fact that to a considerable extent the inmates are 'batch processed'. Although individual patients will have their own regime prescribed for them, and their own pattern of therapy, these individual routines must be set within a wider framework of activity - one in which the patients' daily lives are conducted in lock-step. Their lives are collectively scheduled; the passage of time is marked by the consultants' and registrars' wards rounds, and so on.

Although they may be less regular in nature, life on the ward is also marked by other types of routine work. The patient's stay may be marked by a timetable of observation and management - the collection of urine at regular intervals, the regular removal of blood samples, and so on. Similarly, there is a constant background of coming and going by the medical and other staff. Most clearly observable of this is the activity associated with the work of the various specialist units and 'limited practitioners' (Wardwell, 1963) at work in the hospital. Such practice includes the work of X-ray departments, physiotherapy, occupational therapy and so on. Indeed, on a busy morning the ward of a teaching hospital is a bit of a bear garden: nurses are busy with their duties; doctors are visiting their patients either alone or in rounds; physiotherapists are walking patients up and down; radiographers wheel portable X-ray machines in and out of the ward; porters wheel patients off to specialist departments for tests, or procedures, and on surgical units

110

they take them back and forth between the wards and the operating theatres.

Thus, insofar as there is an observable order of the hospital ward, it is achieved through the formal and informal coordination of the work of the various specialists the grades of staff; the order is achieved through the ongoing process of negotiation of work practices and their timing. (cf. Strauss *et al.*, 1963). Although such order is not always achieved, the smooth running of the ward depends upon the successful interlocking of the various timetables and routines of the various hospital tasks.

In many ways, the teaching that takes place on the wards crosscuts these interwoven patterns of work. Bedside teaching does not necessarily follow the rhythm of the ward. To take a simple example, patients' morning tea or coffee may often lie cold and abandoned on the bedside tables as their elevenses coincide with a visit from the teaching round. Similarly the tail end of the morning's teaching may coincide or overlap with the distribution of the patients' lunches, and so the two activities become mutually disrupting. When the schedules of routine therapeutic work and educational work clash, the entire educational exercise may be threatened. A major consequences of such contingencies is reflected in the problem of *access* to patients. This becomes particularly crucial for students when allocated to work individually with a patient over several days - to take a full history, complete a full physical examination and hand in a written report that includes a differential diagnosis. When they come to visit their patient they may quite often find that he or she is unavailable, and is being worked on by other personnel or away in another department.

I frequently spoke with students who were hanging about in the corridors or 'sloping off' for coffee because 'their' patient was not available to answer their questions or submit to their examination.

> I went out to find the students, who were waiting in the corridor. Two or three of them were chatting with one another. Cross said he didn't know how he was going to see his patient this week, as there was a extremely long list of things they wanted to do to him.

As I have indicated, this could arise from a multitude of hospital routines. Students occasionally went into the wards to interview a patient only to find that they were in the line of progress of a ward round led by the chief of the firm, and had to beat a retreat to the canteen or corridor. For students undertaking clerking the problem of access is acute; since they have been allocated to specific patients, the expedient of sidetracking to a different patient or task is not generally open to them. This, of course, contrasts with the position of the teaching physician. He or she too may find a patient unavailable, but is always able to redefine the work of the session: for instance to discuss patients *in absentia*, share the results of tests carried out on them, or present X-ray pictures. Clinical teachers are also free to move on to another patient, or even to a different illness from what they originally had in mind. For instance:

> Whilst Dr. Shepherd was teaching, Dr. Mayer came into the teaching room. 'We have a terrible problem'. Dr Mayer broke in, 'Mr. Jewson has gone to the [peripheral] Hospital'. Dr. Shepherd replied, 'Oh well, he'll be back in a day or two, and the boys can go round and look at him'. And for the subsequent teaching session, for which the doctors had expected to visit that patient, an alternative topic and a different patient were improvised.

Occasionally, doctors may ignore the disappearance of the patient and conduct the teaching session at the empty bedside. This was sometimes pointed out to me by the students as an extreme example of the contrived nature of some bedside teaching: that such clinical work was done without the participation of the patient. For example:

> When we turned to talk to the second patient, we came to an empty bed, and Mr. Jackson explained that, as often happens, he had been 'whisked away' to X-ray, and that probably his X-rays had gone with him. Still, he said, he still had the notes, and we could go back to the teaching room in the other ward.

In general, these problems of access involve a postponement of students' clinical work. However, the competing schedules of clinical work and education may offer more permanent obstacles to the students. The patient's hospital career may come to an end and all further access be precluded. While a student is working on a patient, he or she may be discharged and sent home, for example:

> Jane Peters had a case history that she had written up, and didn't know whom to get hold of to hand it in. John Carter had also written up his history but likewise hadn't handed

it in. Jane Peters said something to the effect that hers was the last to get done, and Dougie Callan said that he had been unable to complete case notes on his patient, since she had gone home. One of the others commiserated on the difficulty of having a patient go home.

An alternative outcome, which leads to the cancellation of students' work rather than postponement, is the death of a patient. Again, as with the timing of recovery and discharge, the estimated timing of death is an uncertain eventuality and can be an unforeseen disruption of the scheduling of educational work:

> Jim Barnes said he hoped that perhaps Dr. Roy, who was due to teach the clinique, might show them the case of paraquat poisoning. (The case had received wide publicity in the city and was one of a number of similar self-poisonings that had occurred in recent months.) Clay said that the patient had died last week. 'How inconsiderate', said Barnes.

The two features of the unpredictable timetables of illnesses, and the divergent schedules of teaching and other hospital work are sharply highlighted in events which surround the death of a patient. Although the patient's death will inevitably interrupt students' history-taking and diagnostic work, that patient does not cease to be an object of clinical and instructional interest. There is the post mortem to be performed. But the patient may expire at a time which does not cohere with the schedules of teaching, and the routine of the pathologists does not necessarily take account of their schedule either. This can be illustrated from the following case summary:

> The patient in question was an alcoholic, suffering from a number of severe problems, including brain damage. He was now bleeding from the gut: surgeons had been unable to trace the source of the bleeding and further surgery was not possible. The patient was barely conscious and it appeared that little could be done for him.
> The students examined the patient, and then retired to the teaching room with the consultant to discuss the management of the case. At the end of the session the consultant told the students that this patient would last

three weeks, perhaps less. He would, he added, 'make an interesting post mortem. You ought to go along'. There were a number of issues which a post mortem would demonstrate to the students: one, the exact state of the patient's liver, and two, the site and nature of the lesion from which he was bleeding.

Just over a fortnight later, as I chatted with students in the coffee bar, they were complaining that the patient had died the night before last, and the post mortem had been completed the following afternoon, when none of the students could be present.

The unpredictability of clinical time may also disrupt the smooth flow of education in surgical units. The teaching of students must be fitted in with the important work of surgical operations. Whereas physicians may be able to schedule their rounds with a fair degree of accuracy, surgeons may find it more difficult to predict the time that they will have to put in to complete their list of operations. Operations may not prove as straightforward as first thought, and the time allocated may have to be exceeded. Once a surgeon is committed to the morning's work in the theatre it must be completed. Surgeons have less room for manoeuvre in the possibility of sidetracking from the schedule of clinical work to that of teaching. Hence students complained that in some units - particularly those with a small staff complement - they were quite often left stranded with nobody to teach them, as surgeons were unable to get away from their clinical duties when the timetable indicated.

In this regard at least, the scheduling of clinical and educational work presents the students with problems of access both to patients and to clinical teachers. Indeed Becker *et al.*(1961) identify problems of access as the major difficulty facing the Kansas students in their first clinical year:

> The major problem patients present for the student on the hospital wards, then, is to maintain this continuing relationship in such a fashion as to be able to get the necessary information for the job he is assigned. (p.315)

Becker *et al.* do not cover all the implications of time in the wards, however. Hospital wards have a rhythm based upon the patterns of admissions and discharges. The units admit patients for emergencies on a rota basis, each ward having a different waiting (or receiving) night. Thus

114

on, and immediately after, waiting night, the ward has fresh clinical material. As the week wears on there will be a diminishing numbers of patients for students to see, whose stories have not been told and examinations taken place.

Thus the *turnover* of patients in the ward, and the *duration* of their stay also have a bearing on the performance of clinical teaching. If there are many patients in for a lengthy period (e.g. those who are slowly being rehabilitated after a stroke) then the number of new patients will be restricted, and units may even run out of fresh patients to teach on. Such an eventuality may occur in medical units, but is highly unlikely on surgical wards. The mean duration of hospital stay varies markedly between general medical and general surgical cases. Available official statistics for the region at the time of the fieldwork cite a mean stay of nearly eleven days for surgical patients against eighteen days for medicine. Hence there is a more rapid throughput of patients in surgery, and little danger of fresh clinical problems starting to run out. Thus, to summarise, the dimension of time means that not only do students have problems of access to patients, they also face problems of access to new patients.

As I have indicated in this chapter, then, the nature of the social reality which students encounter is not a straightforward matter. While the rhetoric of clinical experience suggests that the students are immersed in real medicine, we have seen that, like any other medical encounter, bedside teaching must be socially accomplished. Furthermore, the successful management of bedside teaching may even run counter to the social organisation of routine clinical work on the wards. To some extent, as following chapters explore in more detail, the reality of clinical instruction is an artfully contrived version of medical work.

6 The social distribution of bedside knowledge

The management of awareness and control of information

One of the basic constraints that hedges round many hospital encounters is that involving 'awareness' and information control. This has been discussed primarily with regard to dying patients and their awareness - or otherwise - of their prognosis. Such a concern is at once a practical one for the doctor and also one that has generated more formal concerns for sociological writing. The most systematic study of the doctor's dilemma and its subsequent working out is that of Glaser and Strauss (1965). They were particularly interested in the ways in which social interaction involving the patient, relatives, nursing and medical staff, is oriented towards the management of awareness. As their main analytic framework Glaser and Strauss employ the notion of an 'awareness context'. They single out four ideal typical awareness contexts - 'open', 'closed', 'suspicion' and 'pretense'.

> An *open* awareness context obtains when each interactant is aware of the other's true identity and his own identity in the eyes of the other. A *closed* awareness context obtains when one interactant does not know either the other's identity or the other's view of his identity. A *suspicion* awareness context is a modification of the closed one: the interactant suspects the true identity of the other or the other's view of his own identity, or both. A *pretense* awareness is a modification of the open one: both interactants are fully aware but pretend not to be. (Glaser and Strauss, 1964)

In the course of their hospital ethnography, Glaser and Strauss trace the interactions whereby such contexts are constituted, maintained or transformed. For instance, they examine the coalitions and teamwork whereby physicians and nurses work together to keep a patient they believe to be dying in a state of ignorance about the prognosis.

The adjudication of the gravity of medical news, and its possible effects on the patient (whether or not the physicians have pronounced him or her to be 'dying'), is an ever-present feature of bedside teaching and clinical work. At the outset of their work on the wards students are explicitly coached in the need to maintain awareness contexts: this is especially crucial in the case of closed awareness. On my first day in the hospital with a group (it was their first day on the wards too) we had an introductory talk which included the specific injunction that students should 'exercise extreme care at the patient's bedside, and put oneself in the patient's place. One does not talk about cancer, carcinoma, tumour, syphilis...'. And on the following day, during one of the introductory lectures, I made the following notes:

> Avoid use of word 'cancer', although you may use it in reassuring the patient that he hasn't got it....
>
> With the recent publicity on the harmful effects of smoking, it is now very important how you frame your questions about smoking. Patients will leap to the conclusion that you suspect cancer.....

Beyond such maxims and advice, the students I observed at Edinburgh did not receive more formal injunctions on the topic of awareness closure. But at another Scottish University, the students do receive such explicit instructions as part of their introductory hand-out for the clinical course ('Notes on the Examination of Patients'). At the foot of the first, these instructions include:

A warning: When discussing medical matters in the patient's hearing, certain words with disturbing associations should be avoided. This is so even if they are not relevant to the particular individual. Such words with alternative euphemisms are -

Malignant disease,
cancer growth   - neoplasia or new tissue formation

Syphilis   - specific disease or lues

117

Gonorrhoea	- Neisserian infection
Post-mortem	- Sectio cadaveris, the Professor of Pathology's wards
Death	- Exitus

The use of such periphrasis and synonymy was frequently recorded in my field notes - although I did not encounter the exotic 'Professor of Pathology's wards'. Clinicians and students alike used terminology such as 'space occupying lesions' for tumours, and 'neoplasia' or 'neoplastic process' for 'cancer'. Students complained that such periphrasis was becoming hard to sustain: the wide dissemination of information about disease processes - particularly malignancy - makes it difficult to ensure that an alternative word or phrase is unknown to the patient. Not only has 'carcinoma' joined 'cancer' as a lay term, but 'neoplasia' is also becoming too familiar for comfortable use at the bedside. For instance, I noted:

> John explained that they were always warned against the use of emotive terms in front of the patient. You don't say lung cancer or use common terms like angina. Instead of cancer you say something like 'the lesion may be mitotic in origin'. He also said that the word 'neoplasm' was getting too well known by the public.

Teaching presents a possible threat to the preservation of closed awareness contexts that have been negotiated by the hospital staff. This is so on two counts. First (and in the early days of the year this was especially so) students may unwittingly blurt out medical information which the clinician may wish to remain covert. Secondly, while students and staff may be aware of the necessity for awareness management, and the students may orient their talk towards such a consideration, the very nature of teaching places great strain on the preservation of closed contexts. The act of teaching must make accountable for the participants (the students in particular) the basic features of the patient's history. As such accounting must be done publicly, talk may be open to the scrutiny of the patient in a way which does not normally occur. There is less possibility of the doctor making some brief, muttered comment and passing on. If a physician or a surgeon wishes to spend any time at all in using a patient as a teaching resource, then the interaction at the bedside

118

is always liable to render the accounting of the illness open to the patient, and thus to threaten previously established contexts. Templeton (1964) touched on this point in his observations on bedside teaching:

> ... the reporting of the patient's history and physical findings at the bedside placed the student in a paradoxical position of trying to choose vocabulary that would both clearly explain the problem to the group but which of necessity would keep certain facts from the patient ... and discussions which took place in the patient's presence without including the patient as a participant inevitably exposed the patient to ... unpleasant focus on the unfavourable aspects of the patient's prognosis.

Thus, the accountability of the illness and the patient's potential access to knowledge of his condition as it is made public, may provide grounds for the patient moving from a state of closed awareness to one of suspicion. Students can therefore find themselves confronted by the problem of how to discuss things with their teachers without spoiling the patient's state of awareness, or causing distress. As one student put it:

> 'When you're asked to discuss what you think is wrong with the patient ... I wish we could go away from the earshot of the patient ... you might say the wrong thing. You think desperately how you can describe the lump without frightening people.'

Hospital patients have been observed to try to elicit information from various types of personnel in the wards. The patient who is anxious or suspicious as to the nature of his or her condition may attempt to pump people for information. If doctors will not divulge what the patient feels to be sufficient information then the nurses will be turned to (Glaser and Strauss, 1965, p.55 ff.) The students who come to talk to them also offer patients a further possible source of knowledge. Hence it is a continuing concern of students to guard against divulging information. Several of the students I interviewed told me that when they were clerking a patient individually they had been asked 'awkward questions'. To quote just one:

> Heather Morgan told me that she had had a patient ask her about her condition on her first day of clinical work in medicine. She added that she had had to 'hedge' and avoid giving the patient a direct reply.

Glaser and Strauss describe how nurses were able to avoid such problems, to some extent at least, by referring patients to the chain of command on the ward. They were able to deflect unwelcome or embarrassing questions of telling the patients that they should ask the doctors about their condition and prognosis. As the authors quote, they would use a variant of the reply 'I don't know, I'm not a doctor'. In precisely the same way, the students can employ their novitiate status as a resource in resolving any potentially difficult or distressing 'suspicion context'. As one of the Edinburgh students explained:

> If patients do ask awkward questions about their condition,
> then it is an easy let out to say that you are a student, and
> to tell the patient to ask one of the senior physicians about
> it.

Thus the students can claim either that it is not their place to discuss such things with the patients, or that, by virtue of their ignorance, they are not in any position to do so anyway.

A problem in this regard arises from the students' infrequent and spasmodic contact with any given patient. Since they have not normally followed a case from admission to the ward, through the remainder of the patient's hospital career, students are not always in a position to gauge what the patient knows or does not know already. Hence it may be particularly problematic for them to judge what to impart to the patient about the illness, since they are not 'clued in' to the previous negotiations between staff members and the patient in question.

> Heather told me that two of them had been talking to a
> patient who had asked them about her condition. The
> students hadn't known how much she knew already, and so
> had no idea how much they could reasonably tell her.

The students' dilemma in this matter is made worse since different clinicians employ different 'rules of thumb' in deciding how much information to divulge to patients. As one student put it, 'some consultants are adamant that the patient should never be told; others believe that it depends on the patient concerned'.

When patients use the students as an alternative source of information they are sometimes successful in eliciting reassurance. It is also no means unheard of for patients to imagine that they are much more gravely ill than is the case, and if they voice their fears, then students can try to put their minds at rest. When illness is not grave or terminal, then students are at liberty to offer information and explanations. One of the students, Alan Pickering, told me that:

> A patient he was clerking had come in after a bleed: the patient
> thought he was still bleeding, as he was passing black stools.
> He was worried, but was unwilling to talk to the doctors about
> his fears. Alan was able to reassure him that the colour of his
> motions was caused by the iron tablets that he was now taking.

When the doctors appear unapproachable, more junior personnel are turned to by patients (cf. Cartwright, 1964). A concern for the management of information is therefore something which students must learn in accomplishing medical encounters. There are, however, occasions on which it is the patients who must take care over divulging information. This is especially so in the case of patients who are relatively well informed about their own condition.

The well-informed patient

Many patients in the teaching hospital have control over a vital resource in the bedside teaching encounter: knowledge and understanding of the diagnosis and treatment of their own illness. Such information can derive from a number of different sources, as can be illustrated at the outset from the following fieldnote extracts: they were written while I accompanied a male student who was 'clerking' a patient, a middle-aged woman.

> Pt.   I pass too little water, compared with other people
> that is. They give you a twenty-four hour collection
> and you notice that there's nothing there compared
> with other people.
>
> St.   What are the water tablets you take?
>
> Pt.   Lasex
>   ....
>
> St.   What medicine were you on before you came into
> hospital?
>
> Pt.   Lasex and Ponderax. The chemist told me they
> were the most expensive pills around.

The student asked if there was anything else in her previous history. The patient replied that she had been 'in surgical' - 'I had a lipoma on the chest'. The student asked the patient about her obstetrical history, 'Were they delivered normally? You weren't cut open? The patient replied, 'No it wasn't a caesarean'.

....

St.   Any diabetes?

Pt.   No, not according to the tests - they've found *something* now - I'll not tell you.

St.   I'll look it up in the files.

Pt.   That's no good - they don't know what it is. I *was* going home on Saturday.

From this simple sequence of student-patient interaction we can identify a number of possible sources of information which go together to form her history. They are: observation and comparison with other patients; interaction with the pharmacists; her previous hospital visits; her previous interactions with clinicians in the course of her present hospital stay. Thus from her previous visit she can refer to her lipoma and from her current visit admission she can herself report on the negative results of tests for diabetes mellitus. Although she cannot offer the student any definitive results, she can alert him to the fact that further tests have been undertaken and their results noted by the clinician.

Clearly, the range of knowledge available to the patient, the detail, the degree to which it is warrantable by reference to medical opinion and theory - these will all differ from individual to individual. Yet we can begin by sketching in some of the relevant features which are implicated in the process of sharing and gaining medical information.

An example of a patient's understanding which stemmed from a long medical history and a close relationship with the medical profession is provided below:

At 11.15 Dr. Lewis came in to take us to a patient. She took the whole group (twelve students and myself) to the women's ward .... We all gathered round a patient's bedside, and Dr. Lewis asked one of the men to begin taking her history ....

The student began by asking the patient, Mrs Gregory, what had brought her into hospital, and Dr. Lewis broke in to tell him that it was not the *present* complaint that was of interest. The student therefore asked the patient to tell him about her medical history. It was largely inaudible to all but those immediately by the patient's head, and I could see those at the back of the group craning their necks and straining to distinguish what was going on. All I could catch at this stage was that the patient had suffered a haemorrhage after the birth of her daughter.

After a minute or two Dr. Lewis asked the first student to summarise the history, and suggested that a diagnosis was possible at this stage. The student summarised his findings, including the original haemorrhage, a history of sluggishness, and poor tolerance of cold. When the student mentioned that Mrs. Gregory had had poor tolerance of cold weather, Dr. Lewis butted in and asked him 'Did she tell you that?' 'Yes,' he replied. Dr. Lewis turned to the patient and said that she musn't 'give anything away'. Mrs. Gregory agreed not to, with a cheerful, rather conspiratorial expression.

The student stated that he thought that the patient had Simmond's disease, and this was confirmed by Dr. Lewis. From then on, Dr. Lewis conducted the group session almost entirely alone, with some participation from the patient and just one or two contributions from individual students.

Dr. Lewis told the group that the patient had a long history and that she had first seen her when she herself was a Senior House Officer. She described to the students how rudimentary treatment was at the time when she first saw Mrs. Gregory. Dr. Lewis said that Mrs. Gregory was one of the 'Edinburgh collection' suffering from Simmonds disease with various degrees of severity.

The patient herself commented on her comatose condition in cold weather, and referred to it as her 'hibernating'. Dr. Lewis seized on this image as a particularly apt one to describe a common characteristic among sufferers from Simmond's disease.

Dr. Lewis talked about the possible treatment of the disease and asked the students how they would set about it. One of the students suggested hormone therapy, and Dr. Lewis said at one time they had treated Mrs. Gregory with

123

doses of ACTH. At the time it had been very difficult to estimate dosages with any accuracy, and the treatment had been very difficult and uncertain. At this point the doctor and her patient engaged in a private reminiscence about the early treatment and its tribulations. The patient exclaimed that, despite all the difficulties, 'Oh, it was worth it ... it made such a difference'.

As Dr. Lewis was leading up to the discussion of the ACTH therapy, the patient kept looking up at her, smiling and winking. I got the impression that they were sharing a more or less private joke about the vicissitudes of that treatment and its hazards.

The interaction between Dr. Lewis and her patient was, throughout the half hour or so that we were at the bedside, very much a private relationship, going on with shared memories. The students took very little part in these proceedings.

This patient's own career spanned a number of years, and had developed in parallel with the doctor's professional career; she had been in on the early development of hormone therapy, and could trace its subsequent implementation from her personal experience. She had enjoyed a status which closely paralleled that described by Fox (1959). Thus the dynamics of the teaching session were affected by the closely cooperative relationship that had grown up between doctor and patient over a number of years. Having gone through her own 'experiment perilous' she had become extremely well informed on Simmond's disease - its aetiology, symptoms and treatment. She appeared to take considerable pride in her position as a well-informed patient and her privileged status as a long standing 'guinea pig' who had participated in the Edinburgh work on hypopituitarism.

On more than one occasion, the knowledge possessed by well-informed patients outstripped that of the fourth year students themselves. Such superior knowledge or mastery of technical vocabulary on the part of patients may threaten the students with a loss of face. It may be felt to undermine their position as medical men and women. Just as it was a great talking point whether patients had called a student 'doctor' or not, the self perception of 'young doctor' could be a precarious one. Sustained by the student's successful production of appropriate demeanour and expertise, it can be undermined by a failure of medical understanding on their part.

In so far as the patient's fluency with medical terminology and information can threaten the students' position, they may be led to discount the patient's competence. Patients were sometimes implicitly accused of using such medical vocabulary without necessarily understanding it. For example, during the early weeks of the year, the students I was with practised taking psychiatric and social histories from patients in the general medical wards. Having done so, they then presented their case histories to the rest of the clinique and a lecturer in psychiatry. In presenting a report on 'their' patient, two of the students repeated sections of her history verbatim. It appeared that she was using a wide range of semi-technical and medical vocabulary. The psychiatrist brought this to the students' attention as a possibly significant feature of the patient's general attitude:

> The lecturer suggested that Mrs. James liked to be very informed on the use of medical terms - she had been able to name the drugs she had been on, had used terms like 'debility' and so on. Doug Ewart replied. 'I wouldn't say she was *informed*, but she liked to use the words'.

Here the lecturer appeared more willing to credit the patient with a degree of well-informedness. The students, on the other hand, seemed less keen to credit the patient with any genuinely useful information. On the basis of the history as the students presented it, the patient was presenting the information accurately. The doctor was willing to give her the benefit of the doubt; the students were not.

In comparison with the general lay population or patients visiting clinics, the patients in a teaching hospital who cooperate in the teaching of clinical subjects are in a better position to develop a well-informed perspective on their illness. Patients who have come to be defined as 'interesting' cases for the purposes of instruction may be visited by doctors and students on numerous occasions. They are not only required to reproduce their history time after time but may also listen to bedside discussions of their condition. Such instructional discussion provides a good opportunity for patients to glean knowledge of their own case.

Patients as legitimators and coaches

I have already described how the patients may be seen by students as threatening their display of medical competence. If well-informed patients appear to know more than the students themselves, then it becomes difficult for the students to sustain a convincing performance as legitimate medical people. Their novitiate status and relative ignorance will be 'shown up' by the patients. By the same token patients can legitimate students' performances. Not only can patients provide students with a general legitimation of their role as doctors in the making, they can also provide more detailed legitimation of students' performance of their work. That is, quite irrespective of whether they see them as students or doctors, the patients can openly acknowledge the successful accomplishment of clinical tasks. Given the patients' position as team members in sustaining the reality of the bedside session, they may be in a position to comment on the teaching session and the participants' competence.

In one session that I observed the students were examining a middle aged woman. They had been informed explicitly by the consultant that they were to examine 'these neurological legs'. There was thus no question of secrecy vis-a-vis the patient, and the patient appeared to be well aware of her condition. As the examination progressed, one of the students tried to elicit *clonus* (a form of reflex) but was unable to do so. The consultant then demonstrated his own technique, and successfully elicited the sign. The student tried again, using the consultant's method. He produced *clonus* for himself this time, and the patient, nodding and smiling announced to the world at large, 'He's got it!' Or again:

Cons. You asked him [an elderly male patient] about his eyes ... you asked a very general question and got an answer about visual acuity ... but there's one thing you must ask.
St.   [to the patient] Did you ever get double vision?
Pt.   No. [turns to consultant] Was that the question?
Cons. Yes.
The patient turns back to the student, grins and makes a thumbs up sign to him.

In addition to such unsolicited, spontaneous interventions from the patient, it also remains possible for the teaching clinician to acknowledge the position of the patient, and to use him or her to evaluate a student's examination or diagnosis. This strategy can be seen at work in the course of the following extract from my field notes. I reproduce it quite fully as it also demonstrates a clear case of a patient with a fairly full and detailed knowledge of her complex medical history.

126

Dr. Rosen asked what had originally been wrong with the patient. She replied, 'I had a gall bladder'.

Dr. Rosen replied good humouredly, 'We all have a gall bladder'.

Mrs. Baxter corrected herself, 'I had a gall bladder removed I mean....'

Dr. Rosen continued, 'Was the operation a success or not?'

'Just before the end of the operation I passed out, and that was me out for three days'.

Dr. Rosen explained, 'As I understand it from reading the notes, she went into deep shock and needed resuscitation for three days'.

There then followed a lengthy technical discussion between the physician and the students on the possible causes of the patient's collapse. This was followed by a discussion of the biochemistry of the patient's present disorder. Dr. Rosen asked, 'What disease is that?'

A student replied, 'Addison's disease'

Dr. Rosen turned to the patient, 'Is that right?'

'That's right', the patient confirmed.

Dr. Rosen asked Mrs. Baxter, 'Would you like to tell them what you had then and have been taking since?'

'Cortisone, thirty seven and half a day, and....'

Dr. Rosen interrupted and stopped her saying any more about the details of the therapy, saying he would go into that later.

.....

Dr. Rosen went out of the ward for a minute or two, and the students chatted to the patient. One of them asked her if she had two specific symptoms of Addison's disease. She told them she had not. 'That is what is so puzzling about me - I haven't got all the right things, or they're all upside down ... I'm sorry I've landed you with all this'.

'It's all part of our education', said Tim Watson.

In terms of her knowledge of her previous history and therapy this patient comes over as very well informed indeed. In fact, given the puzzling nature of her case, she appeared to know almost as much about it as her doctors did - or at least as much as they could claim to be sure of. As the doctor himself indicated, her previous history is not clear, and again, she seems to know as much about it as can be seen from the official record of her previous operation in the case notes available. It seems therefore entirely in keeping with the picture of the distribution of knowledge that emerges here that the consultant in charge should explicitly turn to this patient and invite her to act as adjudicator of the students' diagnosis of her condition - something which is normally done only by the doctor.

In a similar way the patients, as participants in the teaching situation, may be in a position to clue in the students. They may be able to coach the students in their clinical performances. They can indicate what it is that 'the doctors normally do', and direct the students towards relevant clinical approaches. Hitherto I have discussed patients' cooperation in sustaining the bedside situation in terms of their acquiescing to a more passive role: in supporting cold medicine, the patients are normally required to act in a passive way: their cooperation lies in *not* intervening to provide clues to the student. However, from their vantage point of inside knowledge the patients can intervene in a more active way to direct the students' endeavours.

This can be illustrated in the following field note extracts, where patients volunteer information to the student in an attempt to establish a successful encounter with them:

> I followed John up to the female ward ... and joined him at the bedside of a woman, who was sitting in her armchair, wrapped in a dressing gown. She looked slightly exasperated as we walked through the curtains. John stopped and looked through his note book, 'I must make sure which eye I'm supposed to be looking in'. The patient, with an air of exasperation, replied, 'It's my right eye. I thought all this was finished'.
>
> Edwards and Bell both looked at Mrs. C's eyes. 'They normally do that with the light thing', she told them (presumably referring to an opthalmoscope).

The same phenomenon has been noted by Stokes (1974; 24-5) writing on the clinical examination:

> There is ... a need to look more closely at the type of patient who is pressed into service for the examination. Too often these have been 'professionals' who have made

128

themselves available to hard pressed registrars entrusted with the organisation of the examination. Considering the central role they play, their financial remuneration is, in general, paltry, so they cannot do it for the money; it is probably the power which attracts them, the opportunity to suppress a vital piece of history, occlude a physical sign and so influence a candidate's chance of passing; this may occur at a subconscious level and the most chronic professional patients like to constitute themselves as assistant examiners (some of them have become quite skilled).

A number of the patients that students see, then, are well informed and they have control over important resources in the teaching situation. Likewise the chances are that the doctor will also have knowledge of what has already been done to the patient. These contingencies are provided for by the organisation of cold medicine. But if that exercise is to come off successfully then it must pass as simulating hot medicine. Despite the fact that the diagnosis and therapy may already have been undertaken the student's practice should proceed as if this were not the case. Thus in producing the distinctive status of the reality-like bedside teaching session such previously accumulated knowledge must be managed with care. If the patient should blurt out the diagnosis applied to his or her trouble, then the reality like features of the exercise will be largely nullified.

It is therefore a concern in the construction of such encounters that patients and doctors should be engaged in monitoring the flow of information. They need to attend to what may be told and when. This concern can be illustrated by the following field note extract:

> The students had been told to examine the patient's precordium, one by one. As the first student began, the registrar came back and poked his head through the curtains to see if everything was OK.
> Pt. 'Doctor, do I tell them what's wrong?'
> Dr. 'Under no circumstances. If they ask you what's wrong, ask them their names and I'll come back and find out who they are'.
> Pt. 'It's just that the other day I was told not to tell them, but I slipped.'

The patient's apology thus indicates an awareness of the rules of the diagnostic game. The following extract also illustrates the point:

> A female student was exploring whether the patient (an elderly lady) had any signs of anaemia. As she was examining her eyes, the inside of her mouth and the creases in her palms, the old lay chipped in 'I've had a blood transfusion since I came in.' The doctor interrupted, 'Don't tell them too much. You're giving the whole show away, giving away the whole shooting match!' The old lady clapped a hand to her mouth.

In a similar way, the well-informed patient may help the clinician and the students by filling in missing information, based on his or her own condition. For instance, in the course of a Surgery clinique I noted the following exchange:

> Mr MacDonald was teaching at the bedside of a patient who had had her appendix removed. He asked Ailsa Ferguson for the characteristics of inflammation. She listed, 'Redness, pain, swelling, heat'. Suddenly the patient herself piped up, 'Discharge'. Mr MacDonald agreed, somewhat deprecatingly, that yes, she did have 'some discharge'.

These two extracts clearly illustrate how patients and doctors can jointly engage in monitoring and controlling the transmission of knowledge between themselves and the students. Such a joint production serves to ensure that the students' diagnostic work should adequately parallel the processes of real medicine. The encounter is treated in such a way as to reproduce the ways in which the inquiry should proceed - as if the diagnosis had not in fact already been done. In this way cold medicine can be done in such a way as to mimic the nature of 'hot' medical work.

The following field note extract shows clearly how the consultant can set about controlling the use of previously acquired information. In this instance, the doctor established a kind of 'meta-game', which provided the rationale for following the rules of cold medicine teaching. Jokingly, he provided a setting for an interaction in which the patient's own resources of information could be held in abeyance.

The consultant began the teaching session by telling the students, 'Imagine that Mr. Crawford is an Eskimo, who's deaf and dumb and mentally deficient'. In other words, they were not to take a history, but were to proceed straight to a physical examination. As the various students took the patient's pulse, examined him for sacral oedema, tested his eye movements, examined his thyroid, etc., the consultant commented to the patient that he was 'doing fine', and that he was using him as a 'male model'. The consultant then asked one of the students, to examine the patient's precordium. When the student opened the patient's pyjama jacket, he exposed an old operation scar on the left side of the man's chest.

Pt.   'Do I tell them about that?'
Cons. 'No. As far as they're concerned that's a shark's tooth that tore you apart....'

In this extract we can detect some of the features of the distribution of knowledge. Hitherto in the session the knowledge and information which was being used in the teaching session had been entirely the prerogative of the consultant. Now, as his scar was exposed, the patient's personal knowledge was brought into play, and his ability to divulge or keep back this information became a crucial resource in the teaching interaction. The consultant brought the patient back into line by reaffirming his fictional role and so re-established his conspiracy of silence with the patient.

The following extract also exemplifies how physicians may orient their teaching practices to the possibility of the patient divulging the diagnosis to the students before the students themselves have gone through the history and attempted their own differential diagnosis:

The first patient that Dr. Porter took us to see was a lady in her seventies. Dr. Porter asked her if we could look at her tummy. She pulled up her nightdress to reveal a band of sore places round her midriff.

Dr. Porter asked Bell, 'What do you think that is?', and turning to the patient added, 'Don't tell them what it is'. Bell looked at her in silence for some moments, then said, 'She might as well as tell me what it is'.

Dr. Porter hinted to him, 'Remember, the accent is on neurology'.

'Herpes zoster', volunteered one of the other students.
'Herpes zoster', repeated Dr. Porter approvingly.

It must be emphasised that under conditions of cold medicine, the teaching doctor will normally be well informed about the patient. He or she will have seen the patient before, or will have access to the accumulated knowledge about the patient, through discussion with colleagues, clinical conferences, and the folder of case notes. By virtue of such resources he or she can guide the students' history taking and the formulation of diagnosis - and guide the patient as well if need be. This aspect of the teaching situation can be demonstrated from the following excerpt. One of the students had been told to take a history from the patient. After a few minutes of question and answer between him and the patient, the consultant broke in:

> 'Okay, fair enough. Now I would like you, in turn, to ask relevant questions, one question each, trying to get further into his history. And I think it is only fair to say that so far you have not elicited all the main symptoms. What other questions are you going to ask?'

We can see how previous diagnostic work informs these comments. The consultant's advice that there is still a symptom to be drawn from the patient implies that there is some already established list of symptoms. This is available as a topic for the physician by virtue of the fact that he himself has already taken a history, or has a history available in the folder of case notes. Here the consultant's guiding hand was needed further, as the students' history taking continued. Despite the fact that the consultant had intervened, that elusive further symptom was not forthcoming. The consultant therefore turned to prompting the patient:

> St.   'Is there anything else that you feel - symptoms that you get with the pain?'
> Pt.   'No, it's just the pain I feel. That's all, nothing else'.
> Cons. 'Is that actually strictly true? You know, is there anything - I think the question really is - is there anything which is happening recently?'
> Pt.   'Well, apart from the pain I seem to have been drinking, lots of water, milk, things like that.

Because of this, I seem to go to the toilet a lot more
than I used to ....'

Here the physician orients the patient to the possibility that there may be another symptom - that there is additional information that they are both aware of. The consultant indicates that the patient may now legitimately divulge this item of information to the students. Again, his ability to do so rests on the cold nature of the teaching exercise. The doctor can overcome the patient's failure to be forthcoming because he is well aware of this symptom and he knows how it can be elicited. He reformulates the student's question in such a way that it will elicit the symptom that he is hoping will be described. He does this by introducing the notion that things that have been happening to the patient *recently* are what is really at stake (whereas the student's own question gave no indication of recent symptoms - indeed, he could not possess the necessary knowledge needed to formulate it in this way).

What we have seen in the above extracts, and in the previous discussion of well-informed patients, shows how teaching clinicians can manage the situation. By virtue of their knowledge of the patient and the illness, they can organise the flow of information between the patient and the students. They can help to create the reality-like features of the academic exercise by ensuring that knowledge is suppressed when necessary; they can also create the opportunities for information to be divulged when it is appropriate. They are engaged in meta-communication: that is, talk about talk. Stubbs (1975) argued that meta-communication is a particularly important feature of teachers' talk. Teachers are constantly engaged in monitoring who can talk, for how long, to whom and about what. In the case of the teacher at the bedside, he or she is engaged in talking about the talk of the other parties. He or she is also concerned to monitor who is talking (patient or student; which of the students) and the content of their talk. The meta-communication is oriented towards ensuring the orderly exchange of information between the other two parties in the course of the triadic interaction at the bedside.

The patient in the next extract from my notes begins to give the game away, as he starts to divulge to the students a crucial piece of information that the consultant apparently wants to save until later in the interaction. The patient in question was an elderly man whom the students were questioning in connection with what appeared to be symptoms of neurological impairment:

133

Dennis continued, 'Do you ever have ringing in the ears?'
Dr. Porter looked approvingly at him. The patient replied,
'No, but when the doctors use what I'd call a tuning fork
...'. Dr. Porter broke in, 'You're giving away all the trade
secrets'.

What the patient was referring to was indeed a tuning fork, which is
normally used in neurology to test for patients' sense of vibration. It is
struck and placed on some bony part of the body (e.g. the ankle bone).
Later in the same session, the physician was getting the students to say
what they would want to test the patient for, and to perform these
neurological tests:

Dr. Porter asked, 'What else?' There was a period of
silence, as none of the students volunteered a reply.
Finally he reached behind the head of the bed and
produced a large turning fork. 'Vibration' chorused some
of the students.

If we return to the nature of cold medicine, we can begin to amplify
the material I have just discussed. Cold medicine is an opportunity for the
students to practise the techniques of clinical method. Although both the
patient and the doctor may know the nature of the patient's illness, such
knowledge has to be set aside for the purposes of the teaching exercise.
By acting as if previous clinical work had not been done, and knowledge
not accumulated, the members of the clinique, the doctor and the patient,
can re-enact a scene which displays features of hot medicine. The
teaching session can be conducted by the clinician in charge in such a
way as to parallel the routine of history-taking and physical examination,
just as it is done afresh on patients in the acute phase of their conditions.
Thus, although the patients may be aware of the nature of their illness, or
of critical features of their hospital career, the successful accomplishment
of the situation demands that the shared knowledge enjoyed by patients
and their doctors should be suppressed temporarily, until it is
methodically uncovered by the students in the course of their
investigations. These pedagogic exchanges are, for the most part, possible
because the teaching clinicians themselves have prior knowledge of
patients' conditions, prior diagnostic work done on them, and the signs
and symptoms they have presented with.

The doctor's prior knowledge

Doctors' prior knowledge of the patient's condition means that they are often in a position to produce displays of skill and competence in clinical technique. Over and above the fact that the doctors enjoy superior expertise in general, they also have a particular advantage in relation to the patient they are teaching on. If they already know what they may expect to find - especially when performing a physical examination - then they are in an advantageous position to bring off an impressive display of clinical acumen and skill. This is particularly so if they have previously examined the patient and then can simply rehearse what has been done already, and can work back from the predicted result. This is illustrated in the following extracts of field notes, which were taken from the same teaching session in medicine. The students involved where examining an old man who had given them a history of dizziness, loss of balance and double vision. They were performing a series of tests on the central nervous system:

> Dr. Porter asked the students what further tests can be used for proprioception. Grant suggested the Romberg test. Dr. Porter asked him to describe it. Grant described how one gets the patient to stand upright, with the eyes shut; they lose their balance, he explained, as they are normally using visual stimuli to maintain their balance. Dr. Porter asked how one might reproduce the Romberg test in the upper limbs. Jackson suggested getting the patient to touch the tip of his nose with his eyes shut. Dr. Porter pointed out that the Romberg test does not involve movement. He himself (as no further suggestions were forthcoming) asked Mr. Fawcett to hold his arms straight out in front of him and shut his eyes. The patient did so, and Dr. Porter exhorted him to 'Keep them there, keep them there', but gradually his left hand started to waver, and though his right hand remained steady, the left had slowly dropped. Dr. Porter looked round triumphantly, 'I'd like a round of applause for that!'

Later in the same encounter:

> Dr. Porter then tested for the possibility of the patient ignoring one side of his body. The doctor got him to close

his eyes and say which arm he was touching. The patient successfully identified which one it was, but when both arms were touched simultaneously, he only reported feeling his *right* arm being touched. 'I trust you're all impressed', commented Dr. Porter.

Here the doctor had taken the initiative in conducting the examination. The students, despite questioning from the doctor had not suggested the best and most appropriate tests of neurological functioning. Hence, the consultant had had to introduce the tests off his own bat. His tests were totally successful. Indeed, their dramatic success is underscored by his call for applause. Although he would probably have performed these tests anyway, given his neurological expertise and the history as presented, the success of his demonstration was pretty well guaranteed by the previous work that he and his colleagues had already performed with this particular patient.

The clinical tests for neurological functioning lend themselves particularly to such dramatic performances. The patient who involuntarily acts out the signs of his impairment appears as the physician's unwitting stooge in the demonstration of clinical expertise. In the course of one neurology session I noted that the consultant referred several times to his getting the patient to do her 'party tricks', and spoke of his having 'trained' her to do them properly (which is itself a further acknowledgement of the clinical teacher's previously acquired information). However, although the doctor is in this advantageous position to adopt such a thaumaturgical approach, this does not necessarily mean that he or she will always be able to bring them off successfully. The doctors' performances can occasionally fall very flat indeed, if the patient fails to respond as predicted. For instance:

> Dr. Fowler began to speak to the patient, and told us to watch her closely. (The patient, an elderly lady, was fairly drowsy and didn't appear to be altogether 'with it'.) As he spoke to the patient, he gestured to Heather Muir to sidle right up to the end of the bed - so that she was next to the patient's head - to her left. Dr. Fowler spoke to the patient briefly, telling her that he had brought some 'young doctors' to see her. When he had finished speaking, the physician nodded to Heather Muir as a sign for her to start speaking herself. Heather did so, and as she did, the patient turned her head to the left to look at her. Dr.

Fowler laughed, and apologised that this hadn't worked. He explained that he had not been expecting the patient to react to anything on her left side.

The subsequent development of this teaching session went on to show that the diagnosis implied by the consultant's little trick was substantiated. But the point is that he had been able to plan the performance in the first place on the basis of his prior knowledge of the diagnosis - and hence of the likely outcome of the demonstration. In this case the physician managed to laugh off his failure.

I noted that failures in stage management of this sort did tend to produce occasions for laughter between students and staff. Sometimes, it would be a source for covert mirth and sniggering from the students - a sort of *Schadenfreude* and a delight in their teachers' deflation and possible loss of composure. Alternatively - as in the example above - it could be a topic of humour shared between teacher and students.

In the following example the patient was an elderly man, who we saw in an acute poisoning unit. The patient had taken an overdose of a drug prescribed to him to control hypertension - he had thus drastically reduced his blood pressure. Since coming into hospital he had also started showing symptoms of alcohol dependence. He had now recovered sufficiently to be sitting up in an armchair, but presented a sorry appearance, and gave a general impression of being confused and disoriented:

> The patient, a Mr. Wilson, had a black eye, and when Dr. Ewing asked him how he had got it, he went into a rambling account of how he had been set upon by the ward orderly so he could 'keep his job open' - there having been no other patients in the ward at that time....
>
> Dr. Ewing asked him the date, the day of the week, and the year, and he got them all correct. The doctor then encouraged him to elaborate on his story of assault by the orderly. But the patient did not attempt to offer any more detail; or to embroider his story in any way.
>
> Dr. Ewing said that some patients of this sort show 'micrographia' - that is their handwriting gets very small. He gave Mr. Wilson a notebook and a ballpoint pen, and asked him to write his name and address. The patient did this very laboriously. But when we examined it, although

there was clearly evidence of tremor, there was no sign of the handwriting getting any smaller.

Later Dr. Ewing took the students into a side room to talk about the patient:

> Whilst talking about the symptoms of 'confabulation' (i.e. making up stories and fantasies), Dr. Ewing said that he had been trying to get Mr. Wilson to confabulate further about his imagined assault (he had in fact received his injury by falling out of bed during an episode of delirium tremens). Dr. Ewing went on that he hadn't really been confabulating, and he would 'see him afterwards'; similarly, while talking about the patient's failure to display micrographia, he said he clearly hadn't 'briefed Mr. Wilson properly beforehand!'

The physician and the students all laughed at this overt reference to the pre-diagnosed nature of cold medicine bedside teaching. The context was a potentially distressing one - an acute poisoning unit, where a number of parasuicides were being cared for. It was a depressing place, physically unprepossessing as well as occasioning emotional response from the students. Tension and nervous laughter were never far beneath the surface. However, Dr. Ewing's joke at this point came off in terms of his explicit reference to the stage-management of the encounter. His comment represented a glimpse behind the scenes, and of the stage machinery whereby a performance of clinical technique could be sustained. In this instance, nature failed to mimic art and the physician's reliance on his foreknowledge of the patient's condition let him down.

Students acknowledge the physician's prior information about the patient as a resource in demonstrating his clinical skill and producing 'neat' diagnostic findings. I made the following notes after a coffee time discussion on Dr. Burton's teaching style and personality. The fourth year students were sitting with two men in their final year:

> The students had been commenting on Dr. Burton's claim to be able to diagnose a myocardial infarction simply from his observation of cyanosis about the patient's features. A fair degree of incredulity was expressed as to whether Dr. Burton really could produce accurate diagnoses, as he claimed. A senior student said that the consultants often

pretended to be making a diagnosis on the strength of what they were doing at the bedside with the juniors, but in fact had access to extra information which they didn't acknowledge. John (a fourth-year) agreed, and said that when Dr. Burton had examined a patient he'd never seen before he'd been completely stumped. He instanced the 18 year old girl we had seen with symptoms and signs of a neurological disorder.

The patient just referred to had caused a certain amount of comment among the students. The consultant had conducted a teaching session on a girl who had been admitted the previous evening. He had not actually studied her himself, and it appeared that no diagnosis had yet been formulated. Certainly the doctor had no previous diagnosis to rely on. We came upon the patient as a senior student was taking her history. Dr. Burton got the senior to present the case to the clinique. The history was a fairly vague one of numbness, tingling and weakness of the limbs. Dr. Burton asked the girl some questions himself and then went on to perform an examination of the patient. He concentrated on a neurological examination of her arms and legs.

When he had completed demonstrating the physical examination, Dr. Burton commented that the clinical findings were hard to interpret and he had never seen a case like it before. The doctor commented to the senior student: would he like this case in his final examination? The student said he would not and the doctor agreed he would not either. As the students commented subsequently, faced with a totally fresh patient the consultant was in difficulties. He was unable to provide the display of diagnostic wizardry which was something of a trademark of his teaching style. (Subsequently the girl's trouble was tentatively identified as disseminated sclerosis, although when I enquired later this was still far from certain.)

I am not implying that there was any incompetence on the doctor's part: I have no external criteria to discover whether the case really needed to be as puzzling as he made it. Rather, I am pointing out how the circumstances of his teaching session made it a topic for student conversation. Whether or not they were justified in their implied criticism, it provided an apt illustration of their recognition of this feature of cold medicine.

It is by virtue of the pre-diagnosis of patients' conditions that clinicians may select patients for the demonstration of specific features of history-taking, physical examination and diagnosis. In many teaching sessions at the bedside, lengthy physical examinations are curtailed, and the teaching physician or surgeon will indicate at the outset the direction in which students' enquiries should go. They may tell them at the beginning that the patient has had a particular sort of presenting trouble and ask the students to question the patient on that basis - concentrating their questioning just on that physical system rather than taking a complete history. They may dispense with a history altogether and direct the students to go straight on to the physical examination of a particular system.

This sort of management of the teaching session is well illustrated in the pedagogical approach used in one clinique, known as the 'Friday run around'. Here students were given a list of patients whom they were to visit briefly, and examine just one thing about them, or ask them about just one aspect of their illness. Here is a typical set of instructions issued to the student members of the clinique before they left the teaching room to 'run round' the wards. The consultant put up a list of patients' names with the instructions beside them, and diagrams of the wards, giving the locations of the patients' beds in them:

Male, 1st Floor

(1) J.   axial skeleton
(2) B.   had pancreatitis - take history
(3) Thos.R. examine abdomen
(4) Jas.R.   examine ocular movements

Female, 2nd Floor

(1) S.   examine precordium
(2) D.   "   "

A subsequent 'run round' offers a very similar picture:

Male
(1) R.   examine precordium
(2) L.   lesion of left groin
(3) P.   alcoholic - take it from there

Female
(1) H.   right eye

140

(2) H.   Parkinsonism - find out about it
(3) F.   examine abdomen
(4) P.   examine left eye
(5) C.   presented with haemoptysis - find out why

Having received their 'marching orders' in this way, the students split up and go about individually, visiting the various patients on their list. Subsequently they all come back to the teaching room and compare notes on what they discovered with some of the physicians.

These exercises provide students with excellent opportunities for observing the particularities of specified conditions. They normally engage enthusiastically in the performance of these 'run arounds'; they combined variety with the ability to gain diagnostic information (or confirmation) with least effort. This variety of diagnostic game is, as I have said, made possible by virtue of the clinicians' detailed knowledge of the patients which they have already assembled in the course of their routine diagnostic and therapeutic work. In such situations they can, to all intents and purposes, guarantee that if the students enquire and observe methodically, then clinical facts are there for the finding.

On the other hand, for the game to be successful and a satisfying one, then the information should not be entirely obvious, simply by virtue of the preliminary information provided. As has already been described, the process of educational cold medicine can be spoiled if the discovery of clinical information is short circuited. Such short-circuiting can arise also when patients are selected for spot diagnostic exercises. If the exercise is too specific, then the answer may turn out to be more of a foregone conclusion. This can be exemplified in the following incident, taken from my field notes in medicine:

> One morning, I discovered that 'mock' final examinations were being conducted on the wards, and the junior students were rather at a loose end. This was explained to my by Owens, who commented to me that since they had not been allocated any patients to 'clerk' this week, they were having to 'fill in with lesser tasks'. This morning, he told me, they had been given 'little missions' to occupy them for the first hour or so. Owens told me that he had been told to go and see a woman patient and diagnose what was wrong with her just by listening to her voice. He told me, with an air of some disgust, that there was only *one* condition that can be diagnosed just from the voice.

'What is that?' I asked him.

'Myxoedema.'

'What's that?'

'Thyroid deficiency.'

'And what happens to the voice?' I asked.

'It gets low, and slow, and monotonous, and the syllables get mixed...' (he himself imitated the low monotone). '...if she hasn't got that I shall refuse to make a diagnosis.'

He left to visit 'his' patient.

One by one the students on the unit came in and went off on their various 'missions', while I stayed in the teaching room, writing up my notes and chatting to students as they came and went. A bit later, Owens came back, and said in a bored, I-told-you-so voice, 'She had a slow, monotonous voice...'

In this instance it appeared that despite the ingenuity of the suggestion that the student should diagnose from the patient's voice alone, the instruction was too obvious, gave away too much information in itself, and - for the student concerned - undermined what he saw as the purpose of the exercise.

The clinician's prior understanding of the patient's condition is often especially marked in surgical teaching. The temporal rhythms of surgical work mean that patients are admitted shortly before their surgery takes place, and the greater proportion of their hospital admission is post-operative. Prior to admission for surgery, patients will have been subject to considerable investigation; their condition will have been explored before students encounter them. Surgeons' teaching is therefore more tightly focused than much of the teaching in general medicine. Surgeons' prior knowledge is used to set the agenda and to steer the interaction towards very particular outcomes. Those outcomes can be managed in such a way as to ensure pedagogic goals, and to guarantee that predictable diagnostic categories are sustained. This can be illlustrated from the following Surgery fieldnotes:

Mr Ferguson, the consultant surgeon, told us that the next patient he was going to talk about had a history of abdominal pain. When the patient, a Mrs Dalgleish, came in, Mr Ferguson asked Ailsa Orme, one of the female students, to take a history from the patient.

142

Ailsa asked Mrs. Dalgleish what had brought her into hospital. She explained that she had 'had a bleed'. She added that she'd noticed that her stools were black, and that then she'd vomited dark, blood-stained vomit, and noticed more blood in her stools. Ailsa began to explore the circumstances of her 'bleed', but Mr. Ferguson butted in and told her to concentrate on the patient's abdominal pain.

Ailsa did so, and this included some discussion concerning the exact nature of the patient's pain. It was established that it was a 'sharp' pain, and periodic in nature. Ailsa asked Mrs Dalgleish if there was anything that made the pain worse. She said that it would come on if she got 'upset', when she would start 'bringing up acid'. She also said that it would come on for some days at a time, and then abate.

Ailsa reported to Mr. Ferguson that the pain 'comes on in spasms, lasting a few days'. He replied, 'We call this, yes, spasmodic or periodic pain. Not cyclical because it's not regular'. Ailsa suggested that it was associated with 'stress'. Mr Ferguson asked her rather sharply what evidence she had for this. She got flustered and mumbled rather apologetically. The consultant suggested that maybe she had a preoccupation that peptic ulcer is associated with stress, 'We'll ask you about the evidence for that later' he said.

After a few minutues of further questioning of the patient and the students, Mr Ferguson turned again to Ailsa. 'You said it was associated with stress, and you took that back'.

'No, I didn't take it back. I asked her' she replied.

The patient indicated her agreement once again that she got the pain when she became 'upset'.

The surgeon used his own prior diagnosis and management of the patient to set the agenda, at the very outset closing off the student's exploration of the episode of bleeding, and steering her towards the exploration of abdominal pain. It is also noticeable here is that it was the surgeon who introduces the diagnosis of peptic ulcer. No previous declaration of that diagnosis had been made, and the surgeon produced it *ex cathedra* as a candidate explanation for what he perceived as a student error. He assumed that 'peptic ulcer' had been diagnosed and the history reported in accordance with that assumption. There was no evidence for that, and it seemed to be the case that it was his own prior diagnosis of peptic ulcer that drew him to that conclusion. The assumption, in other words, was his rather than the student's and reflected his own prior knowledge of the patient's condition. In the remainder of the interaction, peptic ulcer appeared to be the agreed diagnosis. But it was the consultant who introduced it for the purposes of his own exposition. From then on he oriented his teaching to this diagnostic category, in demonstrating how the patient's history fitted the classic picture of peptic ulcer. The notes of this episode continue:

> The patient said that the pain was relieved by taking milk, and that pain disturbed her sleep. Mr. Ferguson then summarised the case: that peptic ulcer is normally associated with an empty stomach, and people tend to wake up with the pain in the early morning. He asked Ailsa how this fitted in with Mrs. Dalgleish. She replied that Mrs Dalgleish got pain that was relieved by drinking milk, and had disturbed nights. Mr. Ferguson asked Mrs. Dalgleish if she took hot milk. She told him she took cold milk. He commented to the students that this was fairly unusual, as most people perfer something warm. 'So', he concluded, 'This fits into the peptic ulcer picture.'
>
> Mr Ferguson went on to underline the 'typicality' of this case. 'Heartburn. Is this common in peptic ulcer? Yes. Acidity - is this common in peptic ulcer? Yes. Vomiting - is this common in peptic ulcer? Yes. How about these things?' In response to him, Mrs. Dalgleish confirmed that she had those things.

The surgeon, then, used his prior diagnosis of peptic ulcer to interpret the patient's responses and the student's understandings. His prior knowledge thus enabled him to establish and maintain an agenda for the teaching episode. It also provided him with the opportunity to establish the classic symptoms of the condition, and to display that Mrs Dalgleish fitted that classic picture. The liturgical repetition of items towards the end of the episode is also characteristic of a particular style of recitation of types and characteristics.

These diagnostic exercises, with their game-like characteristics introduce us to the theme of the next chapter. That is, the stage management of routine bedside teaching encounters. The spectacle of the clinic calls for dramaturgical skills on the part of clinicians. The social construction of reality in this context rests on a collaborative enactment of clinical medicine.

7   Versions of clinical medicine

As I have already suggested, the overt rationale of the clinical phase of professional training is that the novice is thereby exposed to the contexts of real work. This chapter will explore some of the ways in which that 'reality' is managed, so that certain *versions* of medical work and medical knowledge are portrayed to the students.

Hot and cold medicine

One morning I was standing with a small group of students who had been taking histories from patients, either individually or in pairs. As we hung about in the corridor we were joined by one of the female students. She immediately began to complain about 'her' patient. As the student had started to take the history, the patient had immediately told her that she had mitral stenosis, as a complication of rheumatic fever contracted in childhood. She had, the student complained, 'spoiled all the fun'. This episode, and its connotations of a spoiled encounter, gave me an *entrée* into the problem of social order at the bedside. The feature which emerges in this context is the diagnosed nature of patients in the course of morning teaching rounds; their trouble has been at least differentially diagnosed, and the diagnosis may in fact be considered definitive by the hospital clinicians. Management of some sort will have been initiated, tests ordered, procedures undertaken. Symptoms such as severe pain will have been controlled if possible, and physical signs such as high fever or blood loss may have abated or disappeared altogether.

This aspect of the teaching round is recognised by students. They contrast it with cases that they see on waiting nights. In student jargon, the distinction is sometimes characterised as a difference between hot and cold medicine. On the one hand, hot medicine is seen as exposing the students to real medicine: histories are being taken for the first time and are crucial to the patient's treatment; the illness must be managed and diagnosis attempted. There is a sense of the dramatic, the unpredictable, and the rough and tumble of acute hospital medicine. Cold medicine, on the other hand, is seen and characterised as contrived, involving carefully managed encounters that lack the same sense of immediacy and unpredictability.

The bedside teaching session (cold medicine) is a social encounter which is constructed in such a way as to simulate a supposed reality of normal medical work (hot medicine). I have indicated some ways in which the situation is located in a medical context - and thus resembles the real world; I shall go on to discuss how it differs.

Although a history may have been elicited from the patient on a number of previous occasions, in the course of cold, bedside teaching, the students may be asked to take one yet again. For instance:

> The patient said at one point, 'Half the students here have seen me before, and my history is as big as that.' He held his hands apart to indicate a thick pile of notes.

And

> The patient interjected that she had told her story so often that 'I should have brought along a tape recording'.

This distinction is remarked by students in their perceptions of their waiting nights. As one student expressed it to me:

> I went to three and watched what they were doing. You were there while the actual history was being taken, not listening to it for the tenth time.

And another young woman offered the following recommendation of waiting nights as educational experiences: 'Seeing things as they happen rather than being taught on things once everything's been decided'.

Attendance on waiting nights allows the students to become more involved, at first hand, in the therapeutic work of the ward personnel. They are, so to speak, in on the act. As one female student put it, 'It was good on waiting nights - they *included* us'. Students see things as they are done, and can see for themselves the practical significance of clinical procedures.

The students thus get a chance to participate more directly in the clinical staff's work with the patients who arrive in the wards. Even when staff members are too busy to stop and teach on the new patients, the students whose turn it is to spend the evening with them can still be present. They can look over the shoulder of junior doctors or senior students as they admit patients and perform the initial clinical tasks of diagnosis and management. In contrast with the work of clinical teaching in the mornings, the students also get some opportunity to do things for themselves, as well as seeing things done. They can 'have a go' at such simple procedures as drawing off a blood sample.

Since what happens on waiting nights depends upon the unforeseen and unforeseeable intake of new patients, what the students can actually see and do on any particular night is variable and unpredictable. On the mornings after waiting nights it is a normal topic of conversation for the rest of the members of the clinique to ask those who had been in for an account of what had happened. Often they have to report that little or nothing occurred. Sometimes only one patient was admitted during the hours that students spent on the wards. They can find themselves hanging about with no dramatic events to engage their interest. For instance, I was chatting with a group of students at the end of the morning's teaching:

> I asked Brian if they had been into theatre very much and he said that they had, especially on waiting nights, when one of them would scrub up and assist at the operation. Margaret added that waiting nights were the only time when they learned anything. Harriet interrupted him, saying that *that* depended on there being anything happening. One of the other girls said, 'Oh, didn't you have anything?'

Harriet admitted that when she had been in, there had been no new admissions, and so little or nothing for the students to do with themselves. In an interview one of the male students offered the following account of his first experience of coming in on a waiting night:

> The first waiting night was appalling. It says on the noticeboard that you're expected to attend waiting night from seven to nine. I arrived at seven and nothing was happening ... so we went down to A and E [Accident and Emergency] on our own, and saw the one patient that had

been admitted. Then we went to the pub ... we came back later, but only cuts and bruises had come in.

Although he was complaining partly about the organisational arrangements of the unit he was on, the lack of admissions clearly also limited what the students could see and do even on their own initiative. On the other hand, students may find themselves with plenty to do as patients come in during the evening. This is reflected in the following report from a student who was attached to a surgical unit at the time:

> Sean talked to me about waiting nights. With nine members of the clinique, and a term of ten weeks, since the students came to waiting night three at a time, it meant that they were only supposed to attend three waiting nights altogether. Sean told me that last time he had stayed from three o'clock in the afternoon until three o'clock the following morning: there had been things happening all that time. He hadn't noticed the time pass, as there had been so much to occupy him, going backwards and forwards between the operating theatre and the Accident and Emergency department. He had been asked if he would like to admit a patient, and he gave a pantomime of the enthusiasm with which he had accepted the offer of the chance to do so.

Students can find themselves pitched into the most dramatic and critical sort of medical incident. One student was on the wards one evening when there were two cardiac arrests simultaneously; he found himself thumping a patient's chest in an attempt to resuscitate him. (Although he managed to break some ribs in the course of the external cardiac massage, he was unable to save the patient.)

The hot medicine which students see on their waiting night visits may be rather different from what they are used to from the normal morning teaching rounds. As I have already indicated, although patients may still be very sick indeed, by the time they are on the wards, their most alarming and distressing symptoms will generally have been controlled to some extent. By and large, the ward at ten o'clock in the morning presents an orderly appearance. Although the ward may be extremely busy, the patients themselves are mostly in a quiet and stable state. Either tucked up under the bedclothes, sitting in their armchairs or

149

pottering about between the rows of beds, the patients do not normally present a picture of distress and disorder.

The waiting nights are of especial relevance to students attached to surgical units. For surgical cliniques, waiting nights provide prime opportunities for students to go into the operating theatres and observe emergency operations as they are done. In this way, students see things that are rather different from what they see on the wards, and they can act as informal channels of clinical information for the other students. Not only can students observe surgery on such occasions; they may also be allowed to come onto the theatre floor and scrub up, and assist at an operation. Thus one girl proudly described to me how on one waiting night she had held a retractor for two and a half hours: she had been assisting at an operation on a middle-aged man for a vagotomy and pyloroplasty. She described how she had watched five operations being carried out, and had 'enjoyed it thoroughly'.

Students' perspectives on the immediacy and 'freshness' of the medicine and surgery they see on waiting nights can be contrasted with the managed nature of the patients' conditions that they see on the majority of other teaching occasions. One boy contrasted the two contexts in describing his experiences in surgery; we were chatting together on the coach on the way out to one of the 'peripheral' hospitals.

> 'After waiting nights', he said, 'Mr. Michael takes the students to see the new admissions. If you've already seen the patient, you keep quiet while Mr. Michael plays games with the others, and sees how well they can make a diagnosis. Then you fill in the details - and try desperately to remember which abdomen it was, when you've only seen a little bit of it in theatre'.

This student thus drew attention to the contrivance of bedside teaching periods, and the reality of what happened at waiting nights, when the diagnosis was first formulated. He described the nature of the 'morning after' teaching as 'playing games' and 'false'. One of the female students on a medical attachment made a very similar point to me in the course of an interview:

> In fact by the time we get round to clerking them it's really rather ridiculous because, mostly, they've been treated and all their symptoms - all their *signs* certainly, and some of the symptoms - have gone. And it's also about the eighth

time they've told their story and they're beginning to abbreviate it a bit by the time they get round to you .... In fact I get a *lot* more out of going to waiting nights and clerking patients with one of the final phase students. That's when you get a bit of the excitement of diagnosis - nobody really knows.

Cold encounters

The bedside teaching encounter differs from normal medical interactions in that it is not therapeutic. Specifically designed for teaching purposes, this session is not part of the patient's treatment. Bedside teaching is sometimes spoken of as having a beneficial function for some patients - in terms of keeping them occupied and relieving the boredom of long hours in bed. In that sense it can be therapeutic - but not in terms of the usual processes of diagnosis and management of clinical medicine and surgery. It is occasionally stated by clinicians that there is always the possibility that new information about the patient can be thrown up in the course of bedside teaching and clerking. This does occasionally happen. In discussing with me what had given him the greatest personal satisfaction over the year, one student told me:

> In the second term of medicine, I did take a history from somebody and I found that they had been taking an overdose of some tablets ... and I didn't think other people had got that from their history; and the guy said "Would you do further investigation - because you found that: look at her urine or anything like that?" I found she had (inaudible) nephritis, I think it was. And that was through that, so that was rewarding I suppose in a way.

This was the only example I found of a student's work either in clerking, or during bedside teaching sessions, where his or her enquiries appeared to provide important new information on the patient's condition. On a few other occasions students provided additional information but it did not give important new insights into the diagnosis or management - rather they produced confirmatory evidence for decisions already taken. As one student told me:

151

Sometimes they'll tell you things behind the doctor's back - they'll tell you things that they haven't told the doctors. One time at the (peripheral) Hospital a lady was telling me about her drinking habits. I don't know if she'd told the doctors or not - but she told me that she was telling me on the side because she didn't want the doctors to know. She drank about three or four bottles of sherry a day.

P.A. Did you tell the doctors?

St. Yes. I think they knew she was more or less an alcoholic but not how much she drank.

Similarly, a student spotted something new during a medical teaching round. We were at the bedside of an old man: the session was conducted primarily as a history taking exercise. But one of the students - no doubt using the powers of observation, as he had been taught - looked at the patient's hands, and thought he noticed 'finger clubbing'. He asked the physician about this, and she examined the patient's hand for herself. She agreed that there did indeed appear to be some clubbing visible, and drew the attention of the rest of the group to it. She added that she had not previously noticed that herself. She complimented the student on his observation, but it was clear that this new sign was not important, and in no way modified the diagnosis.

It is an even rarer occurrence for a student to suggest a form of therapy that has not been considered by the clinicians, and have the suggestion acted upon. I came across only one isolated incident of this nature. I missed the actual occurrence, but I was on the ward the day after. When I arrived the students were standing about, waiting for a surgeon to come and teach them. They were teasing one of their number (Keith Foster). When I asked what all the fuss was about they explained that during an out patient session, the consultant had not been sure of the best treatment for a woman patient and Keith Foster had made a suggestion which the surgeon had accepted. This had been noted by the students as a 'star' performance. As he himself explained to me afterwards:

My mother, she approached menopause just now and she's having terrible menorrhagia and flushing - her face all flushing when she least wants it to - and so her doctor put her on phenobarbitone because it reduces the oestrogen to acceptable levels. .... When things like that are sort of personal to me I tend to think it over ... and whenever the question arose of how to cut down the level of circulating oestrogens in this woman, I just thought of phenobarbitone. I didn't tell anyone else that - I wanted to look smart.

Because of this student's personal experience, he did appear 'smart' to the consultant surgeon and to his fellow students. The fact that it became such a topic of conversation and teasing among the members of the clinique indicates just how rare and noteworthy such an event was - indeed, almost unheard of.

For the most part, however, little or nothing is established about the patient that is new. On the contrary, the patient provides the opportunity for the recapitulation of well-established patterns and generalities. There is a common (though by no means inevitable) progression in the teaching round. It often begins with the clinician and the students visiting the patient's bedside, where one or more students may take a history or examine the patient. The talk between the clinician and the students then moves on to a discussion about that individual patient. Then the physician or surgeon uses the patient as the starting-point for further teaching on the normal presentation of such a problem, the distinctive signs and symptoms, similar or contrasting conditions, preferred treatment and management of the condition, and so on. The transition in talk from the patient to more general problems is often marked by a physical transition. The shift in locale marking this transition is usually a move from the bedside to a teaching room, where discussion could proceed. Discursively, the transition is also marked by a characteristic style of pedagogical talk. Opening up a very characteristic type of question-and-answer sequence, the physician or surgeon will initiate the shift with questions like 'What are the most common causes of ... ?', 'How many sorts of ... can you think of?', What if ... ?'

> What would you immediately think of if you saw a man of Mr Richardson's age in hospital?
> While he's doing that [examining the patient] let's go round and talk about the reasons for scrotal swellings....

Thus, in addition to the patient being a participant, or a passive teaching-aid, he or she may also be used as a starting-point for more generalised discussions. The talk thus moves from the immediate context of the patient to a de-contextualised discourse of generalities.

Putting the clock back

In discussing the nature of cold medicine at the bedside I emphasised how it can be contrasted with the hot situation that students encounter on waiting nights. At this point I shall develop the argument in terms of the passage of time in relation to students' contact with the patients on the wards - and again, consider some ways in which the maintenance of the situation may be problematic for the members concerned. When cold medicine is encountered, the patient's hospital career is always under way, and his or her diagnostic identity may be firmly fixed. Yet for the purpose of the teaching exercise the passage of time must be discounted. There may be an attempt to 'put the clock back' and treat the patient as if there had been no intervening period and thus threaten the reality of the diagnostic exercise by divulging this information.

In addition to the patient's and doctor's information state concerning the illness - the shared knowledge about the patient - there is also the fact that the nature of the patient's illness will change over time. Thus, it becomes a problem of cold medicine that, with the passage of time, the initial signs and symptoms of the presenting complaint diminish or disappear.

Patients who are admitted to the wards on waiting nights with, for example, myocardiac infarction or respiratory failure in medicine, or acute abdominal pain or urine retention in surgery, regularly display accentuated clinical signs and symptoms. The myocardiac infarction will be in pain, short of breath, cyanosed and so on. The patient with acute abdominal pain may be vomiting, may display a distended abdominal region and so on. On waiting nights, the students attending the ward will see the patient's distress and the clear indications of their conditions. Yet by the time the bulk of regular ward teaching takes place, things have changed. The use of analgesics, for instance, will mean that severe pain will routinely be diminished. Similarly, the acute signs and symptoms of respiratory failure, high fever, or blood loss will have been remedied by appropriate treatment soon after admission.

> We passed on to another women who was lying curled up in bed with a cage over her legs. Dr. Burton took his stethoscope and listened at the apex of her chest, and then got the students to do so. He commented to Jane Peters - who had been in on the previous night - that the breath sounds had changed considerably since the women's

admission on the previous day, and she agreed that there were certain differences. Dr. Burton pointed out that the patient had been on penicillin for just twelve hours, but that it was already taking effect.

Or again, during the same morning's teaching we spent some time at the bedside of an elderly male patient:

> The patient, who was himself a retired GP, recognised two of the members of the round as the housemen who had admitted him the previous night. One of them described to us that this patient's neck veins had been 'sticking out like tree trunks'. We all looked at the neck veins, but they did not appear to be distended at all.

The abatement of signs presents problems for the clinical teacher. When he comes to demonstrate a point of diagnostic observation, the signs which he wishes to show the students may well elude him altogether.

> Dr. Miller reminded us that anaemic patients often have a dry, red, swollen tongue. He asked Miss Milligan to put out her tongue: it looked quite normal. 'I'm very disappointed', the doctor said, 'On Saturday, she had a red, swollen tongue'.

Such contingencies may spoil the clinician's smooth production of a teaching display. Thus on one occasion, a consultant was attempting to display the elicitation of nystagmus - involuntary flickering movement of the eyes. Although the consultant appeared satisfied that there was some nystagmus present it was by no means marked. In the middle of teaching on this first patient, he therefore charged off, taking the students and me with him, and took us off to another ward and a new patient. He immediately started to test the new patient's eyes, and was clearly crestfallen when this patient no longer displayed the nystagmus he had expected to see. Anticlimax was total. The reason for the disappearance of nystagmus was not apparent. Such problems are especially vexing when the disapparance of the clinical sign is not a consequence of the therapy that patients have received. For instance:

After a lengthy discussion of polycythaemia, based partly
on a run-through of a report of a blood film taken from the
patient, and ending with comments on possible treatment,
Dr. Cowan concluded, 'Unfortunately, Mr. Gower's next
two blood counts are normal'. 'Without treatment?' one or
two of the students asked. Dr. Cowan confirmed, 'Without
treatment'.

Such an eventuality is doubly problematic for clinical teaching. In the
first place, the spontaneous remission of a sign impedes the diagnostic
'game'; but secondly, it does not even provide occasion for a
demonstration and affirmation of the efficacy of approved therapy. At
least in my earlier example, the consultant could sidetrack from
diagnostic signs to the swift and beneficial action of penicillin. In the
present context, even that alternative is not open.

These aspects of the accomplishment of clinical teaching clearly
illustrate the divergent relevancies of therapeutic and educational work in
the hospital. On the one hand, there is the physician's concern for treating
the patient - effecting a cure, or at least palliation of his symptoms. On
the other hand, the physician also has concerns relevant to his teaching,
where his routine clinical work may be in conflict with his immediate
educational objectives. Thus the doctor's 'disappointment' over the
patient's tongue, or the 'unfortunately' in the episode above can be seen
as oriented to the relevance for clinical teaching. The abatement of
diagnostic signs therefore presents a crucial problem in the successful
production of a clinical mock-up. It is hard to sustain the bedside teaching
session as an approximation to real diagnostic work when the physical
manifestations that would determine such a diagnosis are missing or
masked. Therapeutic success can spell educational difficulty.

The development of the patient's career and the episodic interruptions
of bedside teaching periods becomes a particularly crucial feature in the
teaching of surgery, and students' perceptions of that subject. In some
ways, the distinction between hot and cold medicine becomes acute in this
context. For students, the vivid drama of acute work is highlighted in the
surgical admission, and the immediate involvement in the operating
theatre. Waiting nights provide the main chance of students' presence at
such hot situations. Yet it is often the case that *after* this dramatic
intervention, matters go very cold indeed. For, after the operation, there
may be little or nothing of the original lump or lesion to be seen. Often
there is only a fresh wound to observe, and the paraphernalia of post
operative care, such as drips, drains and so on. It was an important part

of students' perceptions of surgery, as against medicine, that apart from waiting nights, there was little or nothing for them to see, and thus reduced scope for undertaking diagnosis.

There is a distinction to be drawn between the trajectories of patient careers as between medical and surgical cases. Whereas in both situations the case passes from hot to cold, the shape of such a passage differs. For most medical cases, signs, symptoms and so on diminish by degrees; even after intensive care, patients may go on displaying signs. For most surgical cases, the intervention of such surgery marks a sharp break in the illness trajectory. The course of the trouble is routinely charted in terms of pre- and post-operative phases, and reckoned in post operative days. There is, in general, no sharp division in the medical patient's hospital career. (Here I am of course concerned only with the 'in-patient' phase of the overall patient career. For cases of both types, the admission to the hospital ward marks a sharply defined status passage.)

An alternative way of expressing this is to point out that the students' contact with patients is typically episodic and intermittent. The bedside teaching session represents one interlude in the course of the patient's career, as it is negotiated over time. (Indeed, it is often seen as 'time out' for the patients - as a possibly entertaining session and a relief from the boredom of life on the ward.)

Some patients are visited only once during their stay in hospital. One of the tasks to be done in a teaching period is to produce an account of the patient's career and the trajectory of his illness. As we have seen, there may be an attempt to discount the passage of time and to reconstitute it from the beginning - by taking a history as if the patient were being newly admitted. Yet, in addition, the relevant information may no longer be retrievable in that manner.

In the light of the problem of the abatement of signs, a further theme can be introduced. This concerns the way in which the clinician teaches by means of a retrospective appeal to his own knowledge of the patient's prior condition. This arises from two contingencies of the passage of time. First, the clinician may encounter the problem of the abatement of diagnostic clues, as I have already outlined. Alternatively, it may happen that, with repetition, the patient's telling of his own story changes. The doctor will have an understanding of the patient's illness, based on previous clinical work, and histories elicited on previous occasions. Problems are therefore created if the patient's history - part of the evidence for the doctor's formulation of the illness - now appears to be at odds with that which originally informed the diagnosis. Changes in the patient's history may simply be a reflection of forgetfulness, as some items are now felt with less salience than they previously were. Also, in presenting their history repeatedly - and, in 'tidying it up' and getting it 'off pat' - patients may unwittingly omit information: information which they hear as irrelevant detail, but which the doctor and students might hear as important diagnostic indications.

Alternatively, the patient may attempt to improve upon her or his original history - and add or subtract information in accordance with what the doctor is thought to be seeking. As Turner points out:

> Conceivably ... the 'repetition' of the therapist's request for an account may be taken by patients as a rejection of accounts given to date., and as signifying that the patient has yet to answer the question, 'Why are you here?'.
>
> (Turner, 1972)

If the patient, then, in the face of repeated requests for the story, should hear these requests in such a way, then he may come to doctor his own history in a search for one which will pass muster as an adequate account. The history is repeated in terms of 'Will this do?', and in the telling of it, it is changed from occasion to occasion.

Additionally, we must also note the possibility of forms of deviance disavowal as patients rewrite their medical biography. Again, as severely disabling or distressing symptoms are less in evidence, patients may come to 'normalise' their condition in retrospect. They may make light of matters such as pain, which previously they made much of, as they underplay the severity of their own problem. Such normalisation may be a stratagem designed to alleviate patients' own anxieties, or to express the desire not to be 'too much trouble' to the hospital staff (cf. Davis, 1961, 1963).

For a number of reasons, then, the complaint as it now appears or as it is now described, may differ significantly from the original presentation. It is in the face of such occurrences that the teaching doctor can invoke the 'in fact' clause. Discrepancies are rectified, and the possibly competing accounts - of the doctor and his patient - are shown to be an artefact of the lapse of time rather than a failure of diagnostic procedure. An instance of this occurred during a history-taking exercise with a senior house officer and an elderly male patient. The old man was very hard of hearing, and was described by the houseman as being 'not the best of historians'. I noted after this session:

> [In response to questioning from one of the students] the patient reported that he had not been having to pass water

many times during the day. But Dr. May commented, 'In fact, he reported frequency during the day as well ....' She also explained that he had been sick the day before he came in, although on admission he did not report vomiting.

In this instance, then, the doctor repairs the discrepancy by reference to the patient's general failing as a historian - exemplified by a further retrospective appeal to his inaccuracy concerning his nausea when he was admitted to the hospital.

The clinicians' use of appeals to what was 'in fact' the case also draws attention to a further consideration with regard to time. As time passes and the patient's hospital career develops, then - in the great majority of cases - the hospital personnel will become more certain of their diagnosis and the appropriate therapy. Tests, procedures and observation, coupled with the results of any treatment that may have been initiated, will normally rule out at least some of the possibilities entertained under an initial differential diagnosis; more specific lines of reasoning will be confirmed.

The distinction between uncertainty and certainty over diagnoses is an important dimension in the evaluation of the hot medicine of waiting nights and 'cold' bedside teaching sessions. When patients are admitted in the acute phase of their illness, the clinicians may not be in a position to state a definitive diagnosis. As time goes on, and the patient's hospital career progresses, the chances are that the diagnosis will tend to become more certain. (It is not necessarily so: some conditions will go on puzzling the doctors and a definitive diagnosis may never be reached.) From the students' viewpoint, we have already seen how 'hot' situations may provide occasions for a greater degree of involvement in clinical work on their part. Additionally, when we consider the pedagogical aspects, it follows that the discourse of hot medicine may be marked by a greater degree of *negotiation* between the student(s) and the teacher. The interaction may take a form which approaches more closely a 'team effort' in arriving at differential diagnoses. These often have to be couched in terms of 'wait and see'; further decision making has to wait upon the outcome of tests and procedures, the efficacy of therapy, or further questioning of the patient. The patient's condition may be clear, in general terms (e.g., respiratory failure) but detailed investigation of the sociology and seriousness of the condition may have to be postponed until after the management of the initial crisis. In any event, the clinician will be unlikely to possess as full a knowledge of the 'right' answers as he will when the patient is seen in the course of a normal morning teaching round. In general, then, the development of the patient's career will be marked by a move from relative negotiability towards relative certainty. The social relationships implied by this distribution of knowledge will, correspondingly, shift from a relatively egalitarian one to one in which the distance between the teacher and the taught is emphasised. This process can be illustrated in the following field notes taken from my observations in surgery. The first extract was noted on the day the patient in question was admitted; the second was made on the day after his admission, by which time the patient has been operated on. On the first day, there was agreement in *general* as to patient's condition, but some uncertainty as to its precise nature. After surgery the position, as far as the surgeons were concerned, was much clearer.

Day one
Mr. Jackson took us into the ward, telling us he was taking us to see someone who had come in during the day. The patient was an elderly man [aged 73], and he looked pretty ill as he lay in bed.

We all gathered round the bedside then Mr. Jackson spoke to the patient. He asked him what had made him come in to the hospital. He replied (with some difficulty) that he had pain, indicating his abdomen. Mr. Jackson asked if he had had any trouble with his stomach previously; he said that he had had 'a lot of gas' over the previous year, and had hiccoughed a lot. The surgeon asked him if he had been taking any pills or powders for his stomach. The patient said he hadn't. Mr. Jackson asked him if he was in pain now, and the patient told us that he was. (Certainly he appeared to be in considerable discomfort, wincing and grimacing as he talked.)

Mr. Jackson then pulled back the bedclothes. He pointed to an old scar low on the patient's abdomen. 'Was that for a prostate?' The patient confirmed that it was. Mr. Jackson then palpated the abdomen; the patient said it was sore and painful all over.

Mr. Jackson told the patient 'It's beginning to look as if you're going to have to have an operation.' He put back the bedclothes, and shepherded us off into the doctors' room, where there were three X-ray films displayed. As we stood around, Dr. Richards - who was already in the room - spoke to Mr. Jackson and they discussed the timing of the operations that they were going to be doing. Mr. Jackson then turned to the films and asked the students what they could see. Several of them simultaneously pointed out that there appeared to be air under the right side of the diaphragm. Mr. Jackson asked what that meant. Somebody volunteered, 'A burst duodenal ulcer', while Redmond muttered, 'Ruptured viscus'. Mr. Jackson asked him to repeat what he had said; he replied that he'd just said 'a ruptured viscus'. Mr. Jackson agreed that it could be any ruptured organ, not necessarily the duodenum. Alan Cartwright suggested that it might be the bladder, considering that he'd had the prostactectomy; it might have become blocked again and burst. Mr. Jackson pointed out that the bladder is outside the peritoneum, and doesn't contain air anyway. Mr. Jackson asked what else it could be. One of the students suggested the gut. Mr. Jackson agreed, and said that he would put his money on his patient having a ruptured diverticulum.

Redmond asked about the patient's pain in his left shoulder. Mr. Jackson appeared to misinterpret the question - saying that it was just derived from the irritated diaphragm. Redmond said, Yes, he understood that, but queried the pain in the *left* shoulder when the air appeared to be under the right side. Mr. Jackson pointed to the X-ray, saying that it couldn't really be seen, but he thought that there would probably be air on the left-hand side as well. He commented that he had asked the patient about the pain in his shoulder 'with the prior knowledge' of having seen the X-ray pictures.

Before discussing this episode, let us go straight on to the notes I took on the following day:

Day two
[In the course of a teaching round with a different surgeon, Mr. McBain] we went to see the patient we had seen yesterday with Mr. Jackson. Mr. McBain asked if anyone had seen this patient yesterday: of course all of them had, and some of them mumbled that they had seen him. Mr. McBain picked on Anne Ogilvy to tell us what she knew about the patient. She got all flustered and was unable to

present a coherent story. Mr. McBain asked rather sharply if Anne had examined the patient's abdomen, and Redmond came to her rescue by pointing out that they had only seen the patient for a few minutes the previous day...

We then went to the side room, where Mr. McBain produced X-ray film from the folder he had been carrying on the ward round. He began by asking the students what they did when they came in on waiting nights: did they just go round at seven o'clock and then leave, or did they examine patients? He was very critical in his manner and appeared to be commenting specifically on the fact that none of them had examined the patient on the previous day. The students defended themselves. They pointed out that they did talk to patients and did examine them, but pointed out that they had only seen him briefly during the day, and in the evening he had been post-operative.

Mr. McBain then asked for comments on the X-ray pictures. Redmond - repeating his comment of yesterday - said that the air under the diaphragm suggested a ruptured viscus. 'Which viscus?' the consultant asked. 'Any viscus'. Mr. McBain was not satisfied with this reply and wanted Redmond to commit himself further. There followed a rather confused discussion. Mr. McBain could see no reason for not believing the air to come from a ruptured peptic ulcer. The students tried to persuade him that Mr. Jackson had told them that a diverticulum was more probable, on the basis of the patient's age, and the sudden onset of the trouble.

Mr. McBain told them that it had been discovered since the operation that the patient did have a history of ulceration going back some twenty years - he had had barium meals and so on. He also said that there would not be air released from a diverticulum. Anne Ogilvy asked why this was. He explained that it would be unlikely for a diverticulum to 'pop' - it was more likely for it to open gradually and form an abscess, which might then burst. Mr. McBain appeared to be totally unconvinced by the students' (admittedly incoherent) account of Mr. Jackson's opinions of the previous day.

When I talked about what had happened subsequently, it appeared that some of the students began to have doubts about what had been said by the teaching surgeon on the first day. They too began to rewrite the patient's history, and bring the discussion into line with subsequent findings in the operating theatre.

This confusion, and the retrospective tidying up of the accounts, highlights the way in which patients' histories and diagnoses can undergo transformation as their hospital career progresses. What is at issue here is not simply that surgery confirms or disconfirms differential diagnoses. What I wish to emphasise is the changing nature of the discourse and the students' position. The surgeon in the first extract used the language of betting, with the emphasis on the probabilities. On the second day, the surgeon was searching for greater certainty in the students' opinions. It must be emphasised that the students themselves were not privy to more information, although the surgeon himself was; nevertheless, their tentativeness was criticised by the surgeon from the vantage point of his own certainty. This is illustrated from the two clinicians' treatment of the suggestions offered. On day one, Mr. Jackson led the discussion from the specific to the general, as he picked up on Redmond's suggestion of a 'ruptured viscus'. On day two, the same suggestion was treated very differently; now the second surgeon insisted that students should commit themselves by plumping for specific diagnoses. Whereas the first teaching session came off as a more collaborative venture, based upon a more egalitarian negotiation of the diagnosis, in the second, the surgeon tended to be much more dismissive of students' suggestions, which did not correspond to 'the facts of the case' as he knew them.

This last example provides us with some insight into the ways in which clinical facts are presented to students in the course of bedside teaching. This forms the theme of the next chapter, in which are explored some features of the social organisation of diagnosis and the perception of signs and symptoms.

8 Reproducing disease

Perceiving disease

In course of their diagnostic work, students find themselves working in a complex field of semiology. It is a field of manifestations which must be interpreted in order to produce a competent diagnostic picture, and to allow for the credible and warranted attribution of some label - that of a known disease or abnormality. The conventional rhetoric of clinical medicine postulates two sorts of data available to the clinician at the bedside. They are referred to as 'signs' and 'symptoms'. Commonsensically the distinction between signs and symptoms is spoken of in terms of the distinction between objective and subjective phenomena. This distinction is employed by medical practitioners, and indeed by sociological observers of medical practice. The contrast drawn is between the disease and the patient's evaluation of his or her condition, between the signs, which 'may be objectively observed and even measurable, such as elevated body temperature or skin rash', and 'subjective symptoms such as a pain in the back'.

Although it is generally recognised that this may not be a hard and fast distinction, it is one which is generally employed in the occupational culture. The distinction corresponds roughly to the two clinical processes of 'taking a history' and 'performing a physical examination'. When the patient tells his or her story, and the doctor poses questions about the presenting complaint, then what is related will constitute the symptoms of the underlying disease. When the doctor turns to an examination of the patient's body - through observation, palpation, auscultation and so on - what is observed (seen, felt, heard, smelt) will be the signs of the disease. Further signs may be forthcoming if additional methods are used (X-rays, scans, endoscopy, etc.) or if less direct inquiries are pursued (tests on the blood or urine, bacteriological cultures and so on).

By and large sociologists of medicine reflected this view in their work on illness behaviour. That is, in Mechanic's oft quoted formulation: 'On the most simple and obvious level, it is plain that symptoms are differentially perceived, evaluated, and acted upon (or not acted upon) by different kinds of people and in different social situations' (Mechanic, 1968, p.116). The literature on illness behaviour is extensive. There is a common interest, however, in the examination of the lay actors' interpretation of their perceived biological changes and states. In other words, there is considerable emphasis on the subjective aspects of illness, as opposed to what is assumed to be an objectively observable underlying disease.

What tends to be lacking in the literature is a complementary concern for the so called objective signs of disorders. Of course, our language traps and beguiles us. Whereas our talk of subjective states immediately invites some consideration of sociological analysis of interpretive procedures, talk of objective signs seems to foreclose any discussion of culturally influenced interpretation, of actors' own understandings and so on. Insofar as such phenomena are regarded as objective facts, then they tend to be taken on trust, and implicitly exempted from sociological scrutiny.

Yet it is clear that what we see clearly now was not seen clearly at other times (or not seen at all). What is patently obvious to members of one culture may remain invisible to members of another. The historical dimension to such perception is vividly illustrated by Foucault (1973). His account of the birth of the clinic begins by contrasting two descriptions of clinical observation, the first recorded in the middle of the eighteenth century, the second less than a hundred years later. The first describes in considerable detail the treatment (successful, it was claimed) of a hysteric patient, who was forced to bathe for hours each day for almost a year. At the end of the treatment the clinician described the 'peeling away' of membranes, like 'damp parchment', from various organs of the body. Foucault contrasts this account with a nineteenth century description of a brain lesion, and the 'false membranes' frequently associated with chronic meningitis. The detail of the description is closely analogous to that of the former account. But as Foucault points out, the second description strikes us as a careful, literal representation of a closely observed anatomical phenomenon. The first strikes us today as downright bizarre, and the phenomena that were listed do not tally with any observable physical state recognised in contemporary anatomy and physiology. But both report direct 'observations', of supposedly objective states of affairs. Foucault uses the contrast between the two clinical descriptions to illustrate the fundamental change which he associates with 'the birth of the clinic'. In his terms, the transformation is dependent upon a shift in the nature of perception, which 'meant that the relation between the visible and the invisible ... changed its structure, revealing through gaze and language what had previously been below their domain', while what was previously treated as visible became a non-event.

No doubt Foucault makes too much of the overall shifts in perception between different epochs. Many classic descriptions of diseases were produced well before the early nineteenth century, and the 'birth of the clinic' did not mark a total 'paradigm shift' in all areas of clinical observation and description. Nonetheless the examples he selects do illustrate the fact that the apparently 'objective' observation of physical manifestations is itself socially organised, culturally and historically bound.

Despite the implicit claim that the clinical gaze reveals openly and directly, students find themselves having to learn how to perceive competently. Throughout my fieldwork on clinical teaching there were repeated occasions when there was considerable difficulty in the recognition and reporting of clinical signs. This applied to perception with all the senses - and not merely the purely visual gaze. This sort of problem was dramatically reflected in the following incident. In the course of bedside teaching, the consultant told the students that he wanted them all to listen to the patient's chest and then come away from the bedside, one by one, and tell him what they had found. While they were waiting to listen to the heart sounds and to report their findings they were to draw diagrams of the 'classic' auscultatory findings for a number of different conditions - mitral stenosis, aortic stenosis and so on. The doctor then left the students (and me) by the patient's bed and waited at the end of the ward for the students to go to him and report their findings. As the doctor left, Adrian Gray commented to us that, luckily for him, he had been working at such things the night before, and so he was prepared for the task. Adrian was the first to listen to the patient's chest, and having done so he went off to report to the consultant. I stayed with the rest of the group. When Adrian came back he spoke to John Finch, who asked him what he had found. But Adrian said he was 'sworn to secrecy', although he did let him copy down his recently revised 'classic findings'. He did vouchsafe, however, that he had been given 'a bollocking' by the consultant. One by one the students completed their brief examinations, bending silently over him, and listening intently through their stethoscope (the patient himself said and did nothing). One by one they left - reluctantly it appeared - and went to explain their findings to the consultant. One by one they came back to the group by the patient's bed, mostly with rather shamefaced expressions. As they did so, and began to compare notes, it became clear that whatever the 'classic' manifestations, the students' hearing was by no means consistent with what their teacher had expected. John Finch whispered to us that he had been called 'a moron'; David Dean reported that he had been labelled 'a buffoon'. They seemed to be rather amused by the dressing down that they had all received. It emerged that while a couple of them had correctly identified *some* of the patient's distinctive signs, *none* of them had produced a correct description of the overall pattern of heart sounds. When they had all finished, the consultant physician returned, and had them all have another listen to the patient's chest, to try to hear what they had been supposed to hear in the first place.

Similar difficulty in perceiving can be illustrated in the following extracts from my field notes:

> The students had been left to examine the patient's pulse, while Dr. Richards went off for a moment or two to talk to Dr. Goode. When Dr. Richards came back to the members of the clinique he asked them to report the findings they had discovered.
>
> When the students were reporting their findings concerning the patient's pulse, there was some disagreement between them as to exactly what they had felt. In particular there was some disagreement as to whether what they had heard was a missed beat, or whether it was rather an ectopic beat followed by a compensating gap.
>
> Similarly, when it came to a discussion of the patient's chest examination, there was even more disagreement. There was no consensus as to whether there was presence or absence of 'dullness' on percussion. Dr. Richards 'took a vote on it', percussed on his own account and used his 'chairman's casting vote'.

One of the students in fact remarked to Dr. Richards on this lack of consensus - asking if they would in time all produce uniform descriptions. Interestingly, Dr. Richards interpreted his question as referring to what was the best technique to use, rather than a problem of the objectivity of their findings.

Even in the apparently more straightforward context of visual observation, things are not absolutely simple. Students often find it hard adequately to formulate descriptions of 'appearances'. One of the signs which students are continually called upon to 'notice' is the complexion of the patient: the colour of a patient's skin is often treated as a very useful diagnostic manifestation. But even in such apparently mundane tasks as the description of the complexion, students encounter difficulties. The following incident was by no means exceptional:

> Dr. Cartwright got one of the students to examine the patient's cardiovascular system. The student began to do so .... Meanwhile the doctor asked James Bury to come round and look at the patient. Bury said he thought the patient's face and neck looked 'rather red'.
>
> Dr. Cartwright queried this, and Bury changed his answer to 'yellow'.
>
> Dr. Cartwright called over another of the students and asked him to describe the patient's complexion. Would he say he looked 'well tanned', the doctor asked. The student agreed, and the consultant wrote 'well-tanned' on the blackboard.

The recognition of abnormal signs, or at least signs that are potentially abnormal, is therefore something which students certainly have to learn in many instances. They find themselves unsure how to produce competent descriptions of what they see, hear and feel. Sometimes the required perceptions escape them altogether. One one occasion I was with a group in a medical unit. The consultant was talking about cyanosis - a bluish tinge to the face associated with heart disorders. The patient we were discussing did not, he said, exhibit cyanosis, and therefore was much more likely to have had a myocardiac infarction. Looking at the patient, the students were quite clearly puzzled, and they confessed themselves unable to detect the bluish tinge to the complexion that the consultant was drawing attention to.

Sometimes, of course, the problems of 'seeing' are those of novel technology. Students, for instance, are not familiar with peering through instruments like ophthalmoscopes, and consequently have great difficulty in discovering the appropriate signs. Similarly, they are unaccustomed to interpreting the 'objective' findings of X-ray plates. Although in this

168

context, too, it is not simply a matter of interpreting observations which are 'obvious', and immediately apparent to all. Students often simply do not see what they should see, let alone appreciate the significance of such observations.

Even the apparently 'concrete' perception of physical contact, such as palpation, can be equally elusive. For instance, during a surgical session a consultant was demonstrating a swelling in a female patient's neck:

> 'So here is this swelling in her neck, and there is no doubt about the state of this - no doubt about her thyroid state.'
>
> The consultant got one of the girl students to come and examine the thyroid. She did so and reported her findings to us, 'There is a soft swelling - with soft edges - not nodules'.
>
> The surgeon replied, 'I thought it was nodular myself'.
>
> 'I couldn't find any nodules'. She palpated the patient's neck once more, 'No, I can't find any nodules' (hesitantly).
>
> 'You're hedging. Let's get another opinion'. The surgeon asked a second student to come and examine the patient.
>
> 'It feels quite smooth in the right lobe, but in the isthmus there might be a discrete lump. But otherwise I agree....'
>
> The surgeon made no immediate comment, but when the patient had gone back to her bed in the ward, he said that we would see who was right tomorrow, when he operated on the patient. He told the students to be sure to see a specimen of the patient's gland.

In the event, when the operation was carried out the surgeon maintained that the thyroid was in fact quite clearly nodular, and that his perception was unquestionably justified.

Students were occasionally asked to produce drawings to illustrate their findings - to indicate the pattern of a pulse, or to indicate the position and size of organs, lumps and so on. Such drawings, as often as not, demonstrated aptly the range of different perceptions which had been made.

The various examples I have provided illustrate the various problems students encounter in producing competent descriptions of clinical phenomena. In the course of bedside teaching students are routinely required to 'observe', 'notice', 'make use of the common senses', 'use

169

your eyes', and so on. The patient is treated as a field, open to inspection which will yield, objectively, the signs which index underlying pathology. But inexperienced students are often unable to perceive such observable 'facts'. On the contrary, they must learn how to see, hear, feel and smell. While they can produce descriptions of some sort - as anyone could - 'correct' perceptions are not immediately given to their consciousness.

The students' inability to produce competent descriptions was sometimes the occasion for fairly scathing remarks from clinicians (as with the boys who were variously called 'buffoon' and 'moron'). The doctors' exasperated comments are reminiscent of Don Juan's supposed responses to Castaneda, and Silverman (1975) has drawn attention to this aspect of Castaneda's account of his education at the hands of the Yaqui magician. Silverman points out how the texts reveal the problems faced by anyone who is learning, or attempting to learn, the world and the self from within another's frame of reference. Castaneda's problem always seems to be this: in seeking to understand his alien, novel experience he never receives any explicit guidance or help. For instance, he is told to discover his 'spot', the place where he feels most at ease. Yet he has no available method for discovering where his spot might be. When he is informed that he has now found his spot, he still has no idea how he found it or what is so special about it. Since his groping inquiries are doomed to be inappropriate, his teacher is suitably derisive and exasperated.

Clinical teachers are clearly more forthcoming than cryptic Yaqui Indian magicians (real or imagined). But in both contexts, the basic problem is the same. The teacher cannot 'have' the experience for the student. He or she can tell the students when they are 'right' or 'wrong', and when they are 'getting warmer'. But there is no way of guaranteeing that students will automatically hear, see or feel in precisely the same way as does a teacher. There are no rules that guarantee it, over and above the basic requirement of argued techniques and reliable technology. Ultimately all the teacher can do is to say 'Hear it this way', 'Feel it soft' and so on.

However, in observing the 'objective' features of diagnostic signs, students have to learn the distinctive ways of perceiving. The consensus of such perceptions - which will warrant their status as objective facts - is provided by the grammar of perception that is shared by the community of practitioners who mutually recognise each other as competent. Students often have trouble in producing competent descriptions until after they have been told what they should have perceived, when, perhaps, they return to have a second or third try.

If students have trouble in producing descriptions of 'signs', then they have equal, if not greater difficulty in eliciting and formulating symptoms. By their very nature many symptoms are hard to describe adequately. Patients and medical personnel do not necessarily have a shared language in which to share the personal feelings of pain, nausea, discomfort and so on. Pain, in particular, demands that students learn to manipulate a range of different descriptive labels which are assumed to constitute a common language between professionals and laypersons (e.g. a 'stabbing pain', a 'dull ache', a 'crushing pain'). One clinician I observed suggested too that they could sometimes try attaching colour labels - an angry red pain, a dull grey ache and so on. On other occasions students were encouraged to look for nonverbal clues which might accompany patients' descriptions of their symptoms. Hand gestures are often held to be very revealing. The characteristic 'crushing' chest pain associated with a heart attack is quite often accompanied by a clenching of the fist when patients attempt to describe it. The sharp, stabbing pain, of, say, a gastric ulcer is characteristically indicated by a more localised indication - the patient often pointing with a finger at one particular spot. One patient was searching for an appropriate description of his symptom, while rubbing his chest: the clinician read the gesture as indicating 'heartburn'. Similarly, students are taught to interpret patients' posture, expression, gait and so on.

If patients are ambulatory, for instance, students are urged to observe the way they walk, as gait may be indicative of balance, coordination and specific motor disorders. For instance:

> Dr. Maxwell asked Jameson for possible signs of vitamin deficiency. 'Weight loss', he replied.
> 'I'll let him off with that', said Dr. Maxwell. He turned to Graham Kennedy.
> 'Tongue.....'
> Dr. Maxwell retorted immediately 'Legs', asking the others, 'Which is more important, his tongue or my legs?' This was followed by blank looks and silence from all the students.
> Dr. Maxwell then jumped up and walked off (much to our surprise). He then called to us to pull open the curtains round the bed, and watch him. Dr. Maxwell then limped

back to the bedside, imitating the characteristic gait of a person with a drop-foot.

When patients are sitting up in bed, too, students are urged to observe them: if they are sitting propped up on a number of pillows, this may indicate 'orthopnoea' - that is, sitting or lying propped up to ease difficult breathing.

Throughout this sort of diagnostic activity students find themselves attempting to perceive the 'right' things, interpret them adequately and piece them together in order to formulate adequate diagnoses. In some instances they are urged to generate a diagnosis on the basis just of particular observations, in snap 'end of the bed' diagnoses. In other instances they have to piece together a more complex semiological field in order to induce an underlying pattern. The 'detective work' depends upon students' ability to arrange the various manifestations into a coherent pattern. Individual signs and symptoms gain their significance insofar as they can be located within a particular *Gestalt*.

The patterning, and the predictability of bedside findings is often referred to in relation to 'classic' cases and 'classic' clinical pictures. For instance, in relation to heart sounds, a senior registrar summarised a patient in this manner:

> She's got mitral stenosis, this woman. She's got absolutely classic signs of mitral stenosis. Don't worry too much if you didn't hear it ... I think she'll be gone [discharged] on Monday I'm afraid.

The doctor's regret suggested that they would be losing a particularly 'good' example, and that students would have little chance of returning to listen to the patient's chest once more. Similarly, in the context of interpreting X-rays of the small bowel, a surgeon remarked, 'If you saw this patient, you might see the classic step-ladder effect'. That is, a visible and palpable 'corrugated' effect in the abdomen.

The description of pain - in this instance its location - illustrates this as well. A student was taking a history from a middle aged woman:

> Anne asked, 'We know you had some pain: where was it?'
> The patient indicated a spot. 'Just here. You can put your finger on it'. She indicated the spot by digging in her index finger.

172

Mr. Fuller, the consultant surgeon, turned to the other students and asked them where that was. One volunteered the answer, 'the epigastrium'. The surgeon asked for a more precise definition.

'Just right of the mid line', the student suggested. Mr. Fuller looked at the patient's tummy, 'Just about mid line, I'd say. Visceral pain always occurs in the mid line. It's pretty classic. Foregut pain occurs in the epigastrium, mid gut pain occurs in the umbilical area, lower gut pain in the lower abdomen....'

Here the surgeon appeared to be insisting that the location of the referred pain, which appeared to the students (and to me) to be to the right, fitted the classic picture, while he filled out and elaborated that classic pattern.

In these various ways, then, students are not merely required to 'notice' and remark upon isolated phenomena. Such manifestations are held to make sense - indeed, are worthy of note - only in the context of a *Gestalt*. By and large, the signs and symptoms add up to a significant picture in the context of some overall pattern - a pattern, moreover, which can be matched to some well established type of disease.

Normal diseases

Bedside teaching is an organised way for the display of clinical methods in reproducing the relevant clinical 'facts of the case'. We need, therefore, to consider what is really meant by a 'case'. The documentary method (Garfinkel, 1967) that doctors and medical students employ is a twofold process. There are two levels of interpretation involved in the production of a diagnosis: they are closely and dialectically related. In the first instance it is the task of medical investigators to treat signs and symptoms as indicators of underlying physiological conditions. Though not always successful, they try to relate these indices in order to read off a coherent diagnosis, indicating the presence of an identifiable illness, disorder or syndrome. At the second level, the patient's condition is itself an 'index' or a 'case' of the disease in question. It is understood in the light of what is known about the typical onset and course of the illness under normal circumstances.

For the purpose of clinical education, then, the exercise does not simply consist in the observation and diagnosis of the patient's presenting complaint. It should also provide occasion for students to learn about 'the disease' in question, and related conditions. That is, normal disease is invoked.

By using the term 'normal disease' I deliberately parallel the notion of 'normal crimes' (Sudnow, 1965). Sudnow describes how American Public Defenders (PDs) construct typologies of offences and the people most likely to commit them. As Sudnow puts it:

> He learns to speak knowledgeably of 'burglars', 'petty thieves', 'drunks', 'rapists', 'narcos' etc., and to attribute to them personal biographies, modes of usual criminal activity, criminal histories, psychological characteristics, and social backgrounds.

Similarly, the PD constructs an ecological understanding of offences - that is a sense of where crimes are likely to occur. Hence what Sudnow calls 'normal crimes' are:

> those occurrences whose typical features, e.g., the ways they usually occur and the characteristics of persons who commit them (as well as the typical victims and typical scenes), are known and attended to by the PD. For any of a series of offense types the PD can provide some form of proverbial characterization.

Thus the relationship between 'the facts of the case' and what is 'normal' is an important practical problem for the public defendant, and on his or her interpretation rests the treatment of the case.

The medical practitioner is likewise engaged in matching the observed characteristics of a presenting case to normal diseases. On the determination of the normal illness depends the expected course and outcome of the disorder and the treatment of choice. This can be illustrated in the following report of a teaching period, during which the physician in charge attempted to demonstrate that the patient displayed the features of normal disease.

> Dr. Mayo took us downstairs to the women's ward: he led us into the teaching room and sent two 'strong men' to go and bring in the patient's bed from the ward....

174

Dr. Mayo then went and brought the patient himself. As she came in he told us that he had interrupted her physiotherapy to bring her to be taught on.

The patient sat up on the bed, and we all got chairs and sat round the bed. 'Who don't we pick on?' asked Dr. Mayo, looking round the group of students - and decided to ask Hilary Morris to begin by taking a history.

The patient interjected that she had told her story so often that, 'I should have brought along a tape recording'. (She did not however seem to resent participating in the teaching session, and was very cheerful.) Hilary asked her what had made her first come into hospital.

'I'll start right from the beginning,' the patient began, and Hilary encouraged her to do so.

The patient described how she had woken up one morning with a badly-swollen toe-joint, which was very painful.

Dr. Mayo quickly broke in and asked Watson if this rang any bells for him: Watson prevaricated, and said there were 'several possibilities'. Finally he suggested gout. 'What causes gout?' asked Dr. Mayo. Watson replied, 'Formerly it was port'. 'Do you really believe that?' Watson remained silent, looked puzzled. Carpenter said it was mostly caused by drugs. Dr. Mayo agreed that it was 'iatrogenic'. He described briefly that modern diuretics (which, he added, one uses a lot) lead to accumulations of uric acid. Watson interrupted and asked what was exchanged for the uric acid. Dr. Mayo said he wasn't sure: he suggested that for next Monday Watson read up on the effects of diuretics.

The patient then continued her story, and went on to say that her family doctor had told her it was 'a case for the orthopaedic'. Amongst other things 'the orthopaedic' said they could cut out the joint, but she had said 'I'll let well alone and keep my joint'.

The patient had then developed a 'tingling', and pain in her right hand: she had previously caught her hand in a door, and she thought the discomfort might be connected with that. She said that the tingling condition in her hand had been diagnosed as 'something internal' - and she added, she was sorry, she couldn't remember more accurately than that.

Dr. Mayo turned to the students and asked them to 'translate' what she had been trying to say. One of the students volunteered that it might be 'carpal tunnel syndrome'.

Dr. Mayo summarised this condition briefly. Watson jumped in with an objection to his description - 'Isn't it usually the median nerve?' Dr. Mayo looked slightly annoyed and pointed out that he had corrected himself when he had said it was the ulnar nerve, and had said it was the median the second time.

Dr. Mayo said to the patient, 'You had trouble with your shoulder too, didn't you?', and she agreed that she had had trouble. All this time Dr. Mayo had the patient's case notes with him and he constantly referred to them in bringing out the patient's history.

The patient also volunteered that she now had a painful and swollen knee. Dr. Mayo commented that the hand might have been blamed on something else, but now we had a shoulder and a knee as well, 'We definitely have a polyarthritis'. It was, he added, 'a very typical story'.

The patient volunteered that she gained relief in her hands by soaking them in hot water, and Dr. Mayo commented to Hilary Morris, 'This is the basis of the therapy, isn't it?' 'Hmmmm', she agreed, nodding.

'What is it?' Dr. Mayo continued. But Hilary in fact appeared not to know. There was no response from any of the others in the group, and Dr. Mayo told them that the treatment was with hot paraffin wax - which he described briefly.

Dr. Mayo summed up some aspects of the case, and in doing so made a mistake in the timing of the history - her visit to the orthopaedic specialists. The patient corrected him. 'Sorry, I've got the story wrong', and Dr. Mayo hastily referred to the case notes to correct his summary.

Dr. Mayo then turned to the students, 'What are you thinking of?'

Hilary Morris - 'Nothing'.

'Well, what diseases of the joints do you know?'

'Rheumatoid arthritis', Hilary suggested.

Another of the students offered 'Osteoarthritis', but added that he wasn't sure of the difference between osteoarthritis and rheumatoid arthritis, as he'd never seen a case of osteoarthritis.

Dr. Mayo then wrote the following schema on the blackboard:

	Osteo	Rheumatoid
Age	60+	40+
Joints	Big	Hand/Small
General Condition	Well	Unwell

Dr. Mayo then read off the patient's history against these categories. 'As for age' he began, 'the patient said she was 53, she's equal on that'.

'That's me being difficult', put in the patient.

When it came to sex and the joints affected, Dr. Mayo said that rheumatoid arthritis seemed to be indicated. When it came to the final category - the patient's general health, the pattern seemed less clear. 'When you came in, you said you hadn't been feeling well, and had been losing your appetite'. The patient replied that she *hadn't* felt unwell. Dr. Mayo persisted, and said that she had been sweating rather: she countered that she had had sweats for many years past. Dr. Mayo said she had had a poor appetite, and the patient replied that she had 'never been a big eater'.

Dr. Mayo left the patient protesting once more that she hadn't felt ill, and hadn't had any headaches or anything .... Dr. Mayo referred to the case notes: 'In fact she had a pyrexia when she came in, a spiky temperature ....'

Dr. Mayo then went on to a discussion of a number of haematological points, and he said that the presence of a changed ESR 'would be nice'.

Dr. Mayo and the students went on to examine the patient's right knee, which had been swollen and painful according to her history. Dr. Mayo asked Carpenter to tell us what he saw. He immediately started to palpate the knee: Dr. Mayo told him, gently and in a pleasant tone of voice, that he had told him to tell us what he *saw*.

When Carpenter did come to palpate the knee, Dr. Mayo asked him if he could detect any fluid in the knee, and Carpenter replied that he didn't know how to test for fluid.

Dr. Mayo explained how to squeeze the region of the patella, and then try to bounce the patella up and down on the bone underneath, when one gets the sensation of fluid underneath. However, when he tried to do it himself, he was unable to produce the right effect. 'That's me being awkward again', said the patient, with a rather satisfied little smile.

This extended summary illustrates a number of features involved in assembling the diagnosis. Throughout the interaction the clinician who was conducting the teaching made reference to the normal features of the case. Indeed, his first summary of the patient's history was that it was 'a very typical story'. The patient herself, on the other hand, seemed to orient herself to the *particularity* of her case - or so I interpret her rather self-satisfied interjections on her being 'awkward' when she appeared not to 'fit' the doctor's classifications. This is an example of how, in producing normal crimes and normal diseases, practitioners proceed by discounting the particularities and idiosyncracies of the case in the course of formulating its typicality.

This aspect of the physician's work in defining the patient as a typical case of rheumatoid arthritis can be seen in his simple classification of osteo- and rheumatoid arthritis. The schematic device presented a series of decision rules for distinguishing between the normal onset and presentation of the two conditions. Yet the implementation of those decisions in practice turned out to be problematic.

In the course of clinical teaching there is a constant tension between definitions of normal disease and the particularities of individual patients' presenting complaints. Students need to be able to learn the typical course and appearance of any given illness, despite deviations from the normal in patients they see. Clinicians therefore make repeated references to possible mis-matches between text-book descriptions of conditions and their presentation.

For instance, during one period of medical teaching, I noted the following sequence of comments which illustrate the use of typical formulations as a device for generating normal expectations, and distinctions between type and presenting case.

Dr.　He's as hyperthyroid as they come...what in his history is not quite typical - about his weight loss? (Pause - no reply from the students.) His appetite should be increased - in fact he's off his food.

Dr.	What about the CVS - what would you expect there?
St.	Tachycardia - bounding rhythm.
Dr.	What rhythm could you sometimes get?
St.	Galloping rhythm.
Dr.	Well, you could.
St.	Atrial fibrillation ....
	.....
Dr.	Now in severe thyrotoxicosis - I've never seen it - but there are two signs that the text books give. There's thyroid acropathy - it's like finger clubbing. You'd need to be in an endocrinology unit to see it ....

Here the physician's reference to a typical indication of the illness that is not present in the case in question is parallelled by his closing reference to 'text book' signs which are not routinely present in many cases. In both instances the clinician alerts the students to the problematic nature of the relationships between typifications and instances of illness. In both instances, the students need to 'go beyond' the indications of concrete presentations to read into them the indications of normal presentations. It is the availability of such typifications that informs a wide range of teaching exchanges at the bedside.

The obverse of the treatment of 'normal' illness and textbook knowledge is the contingency that these typifications may fail to include items of practical use in concrete contexts of diagnosis and treatment. In the following extract, a physician comments on the gap between 'theory' and practice in the context of cardiology. He had asked the students to draw diagrams illustrating the 'classic' heart sounds associated with various forms of impairment of the heart. In the teaching room the physician went through the diagrams that the students had produced.

Dr. Maxwell began, 'Right, mitral incompetence'. He went over to one of the students, 'What have you drawn? Let me see. First heart sound. Yes, reduced heart sound.' (He draws on the chalkboard.) 'True or false? The books are wrong. Every book I've seen draws a murmur to the second sound and stops it there. The great thing about mitral incompetence is, the second sound is buried in the murmur.'

The contrast between text-book rules and rules in use in the context of clinical teaching can be indicated by reference to the notion of 'routine'. Routine is an important organising principle in teaching and learning clinical procedures. The elicitation of a history and its documentation and the performance of a physical examination of a patient should, students are told, be done according to a well worked out 'routine'. That is, it should be done systematically and methodically, following a number of steps in sequence.

Yet it is clear that investigations of inordinate length are not the normal state of affairs that competent doctors acknowledge as correct. While such an approach might be defensible as 'painstaking', it is not normally a practical way of setting about getting clinical work done. Time is not available for such methods to be worked through completely in all cases. The experienced worker demonstrates ability and competence by producing a history and examination in a way which does not conform to a literal adherence to the routine. Students are therefore confronted with two aspects of practical rule use: that the symptoms must be mastered and followed, but also that experienced following of the rules implies an apparent 'breaking' of the rules. The routine is, in the last analysis, 'honoured in the breach' by the 'experienced' practitioner.

Clinicians present the students with this dual nature of clinical procedure. For example:

> The patient was an old man of seventy who was suffering from severe myocardial failure. Dr. Shaw elicited a history from him for our benefit. The patient had been a road crossing 'lollipop man' .... He had come into hospital this time because he was suffering a severe pain in his chest. Dr. Shaw questioned him further about the pain, and any other symptoms .... Dr. Shaw probed with further questions about the pain: had it moved into the neck or arm? The old man reported that it had not moved.
>
> .....
>
> Asked for his previous history, the patient said that the only other illness he had had was when he had come into hospital that January: he had had pain in his calves, and he told us that this had been a 'coronary thrombosis'. Dr. Shaw did not follow this up at the time.
>
> .....

During the course of the history, Dr. Shaw stopped and realised that he had not demonstrated getting basic information - the patient's name, age and so on. He then produced the patient's charts from the foot of the bed and read off some of the basic facts about the patient.

.....

After further questioning the patient, Dr. Shaw took us outside and we stood in the corridor. One of the students pointed out that Dr. Shaw had forgotten to ask if there has been any oedema. The doctor agreed that he had forgotten that. Dr. Shaw then referred to the January admission. The patient had told us today that he had had a coronary thrombosis which had been a 'pain in his leg'. In fact Dr. Shaw told us, the old man had had a severe cardiac failure and had 'died'; but he had no memory of his previous attack, apart from pain in the hardened arteries in his leg. Dr. Shaw pointed out that he had not wanted to remind the patient of that, or let him know that he had died on that occasion.

This extract further illustrates two aspects already alluded to: the preservation of 'closed awareness', and the clinician's invocation of 'in fact' clauses in reconstructing the patient's history. It also illustrates how a physician may not stick slavishly to the systematic, sequential ordering of history taking, as specified in 'official' rubrics. Indeed, after the particular session, the students themselves referred to this. They remarked the contrast between what they had just witnessed and the advice they had themselves been given in introductory lectures on clinical method. They expressed disappointment that Dr. Shaw had been 'so unsystematic' in his approach to the patient.

Indetermination and technicality

Hitherto I have been trying to indicate how clinical work is organised according to two complementary principles. On the one hand, the construction of teaching encounters can be seen as a device for the reproduction of knowledge of which the students and the clinicians can be *sure* and certain: that is, the reproduction of warranted clinical 'facts'. On the other hand, the production of such factual accounts depends upon personal 'experience' in interpreting the rules of clinical procedure. These twin aspects of the production and reproduction of medical knowledge have been examined by Jamous and Peloille (1970), who apply the two principles in a general account of occupations - based upon what they term the ratio between Indetermination and Technicality (see also Atkinson, Reid and Sheldrake, 1977).

By 'Technicality' is meant those aspects of professional work which are susceptible to codification in terms of explicit, public rules, procedures and techniques. The 'technical' aspects of professional work are those procedures which can (at least, hypothetically) be expressed in a precise list of unambiguous specifications. 'Indetermination', on the other hand, refers to those varieties of 'tacit' and private knowledge which are not susceptible to such specification. It is not made explicit, and remains untranslatable into precisely formulated rules or prescriptions.

There is therefore a difference between the mode of transmission of such types of knowledge, and in the relationship of the worker (or teacher) to the knowledge itself. In the case of 'technical' modes of knowledge, transmission could be based upon 'mechanical' reproduction, unaltered from generation to generation and from place to place. The sole criterion for success would be complete mastery of the relevant techniques, on the basis of rote learning, locomotor coordination and so on. Such cultural reproduction could be achieved in a completely impersonal way. The transmission of indeterminate knowledge would depend upon 'example', and the observation of a practitioner by the trainee. The novice would have to 'pick up' such knowledge rather than being taught it explicitly. Technical knowledge would depend on impersonal criteria, while 'indeterminate' expertise would depend upon less readily definable and accountable criteria. In Jamous and Peloille's terminology, indeterminate knowledge thus becomes located in personal attributes (or 'virtualities') of the producer himself - who is thus an 'owner' of the means of production and reproduction, rather than simply a user of them.

Now Jamous and Peloille do not claim that occupations can be classified or understood simply in terms of indetermination or technicality alone. Rather they argue that occupations are marked by a mixture of explicit and implicit expertise, by publicly available techniques and private rules of thumb. What they employ is the *ratio* of Technicality to Indetermination as a device for the classification and understanding of occupations and their work. They express the core of their arguments in this way:

The I/T ratio expressed the possibility of transmitting by means of apprenticeship, the mastery of intellectual or material instruments and to achieve a given result. This makes it possible to appreciate the limits to this transmissibility; i.e. the part played in the production process by 'means' that can be mastered in the form of rules (T), in proportion to the means that escape rules and, at a given historical moment, are attributed to virtualities of producers (I).

Although Jamous and Peloille begin their argument by setting aside any 'absolutist' definition of the 'professions' (such as trait theories) implicitly, they use the I/T ratio to reintroduce 'the professions' in a somewhat different guise:

The occupations and activities which concern us are the ones which lie on that sector of the dimension where the I/Ts are usually high. The sector does not include all occupations nor only the occupations usually called 'professions'.

Nevertheless, they confine their remarks to 'professions' and do not indicate what other occupations might fall in this 'sector'; it is also implied that a high I/T ratio is a common attribute of those occupations normally designated as professional.

There are a number of shortcomings in the approach advocated by Jamous and Peloille. They are highly ambivalent as to whether the indetermination and technicality to which they refer are to be seen as 'objective' attributes of an occupational group and their work, or whether they constitute claims professed by occupational groups - that is, they are occupational *ideologies*. The central problem in Jamous and Peloille's use of the I/T ratio can be highlighted by reference to my previous comments on competent rule use. They are in error in trying to separate out the two aspects; all rule use implies an interpretative ability on the part of the rule user, and such interpretive competence is not spelled out in the formulation of the rules itself (Zimmerman, 1970; Emerson and Pollner, 1978). However much the rules of procedure may be codified, the concrete application of the spirit of the rules depends upon 'tacit' understandings. What we refer to as a 'knack' or 'flair' or 'experience' refers to such competence in the application of interpretive procedures in the production and reproduction of knowledge. Hence Jamous and

Peloille's dichotomy is a false one: what they treat as two independent factors in their I/T ratio are inextricably intertwined.

On the other hand, it is possible that the notions of indetermination and technicality constitute a *rhetoric* in which are couched claims concerning professional work and expertise. From this point of view one might inspect how varieties of knowledge are warranted by practitioners by reference to the two principles of production and reproduction.

The language of indetermination is a language of personal knowledge. The language of 'experience' is the common currency of a stratified and segmented occupation. It is congruent with segmentation since it relies on differences in personal experience, the distinctiveness of concrete occasions, of practice and the diversity of individual careers. 'Tacit' knowledge depends upon the consensus of discrete groups with shared occupational ideologies and biographies. The rhetoric of 'experience' is also that of a stratified occupation. It emphasises a view of socialisation and expertise founded upon a lengthy period of induction in the 'mysteries' and arcane knowledge of the occupation: in the course of a practitioner's unfolding career. Hence expertise is only to be guaranteed by seniority and length of 'experience'. However well-informed a young practitioner may be, and whatever the level of his or her technical learning, it still requires the accumulation of 'experience' to transform him into a fully competent practitioner. As Jamous and Peloille themselves emphasise, the 'apprenticeship' approach to socialisation, and its reliance upon an apostolic transmission of knowledge from practitioner to apprentice, is predicated on the congruence between the stratification and segmentation of the profession. If the rhetoric of technicality is expressive of the common knowledge, and publicly accountable expertise of the profession, then that of 'indetermination' ensures the non accountability and autonomy of the profession, and of segments within it.

In the course of clinical teaching, appeal is often made to 'experience' and 'judgement'. Such knowledge is treated as personal and therefore as less technical or determinate than the prescriptions of 'science' and the formulations of text books. In contrast to the context free, universalistic connotations of 'science', experience is a personal matter, dependent on the biography of the clinician. The quality of 'experience' gained depends, for example, on *where* one is trained and has practised, *with whom* one has been a doctor, and *when*. In the course of his or her career, the competent clinician amasses a stock of relevant experience to draw on.

The following extracts from my field notes illustrate how clinicians may make appeals to experience in decision making on diagnosis and patient management. For instance, in the first extract, the teaching physician alerts the students to personal experience in therapy - and how the locale of one's treatment and practice is a major factor in clinicians' adoption of therapeutic measures:

> They discussed the problems of high blood pressure and reducing it. Dr. Cowan told us that on admission the patient had a palpable fourth heart sound, and they had been afraid he'd go into failure. 'The question is', he said, 'What drug do you use to reduce blood pressure?' The students suggested a number of possible treatments, and Dr. Cowan commented, 'You get used to one drug. Propranadol is used a lot in Edinburgh'.

The same consideration is apparent in the consultant surgeon's pronouncement in the following extract. The remarks were noted in a tutorial class on breast cancer. The surgeon had explained to the clinique the difference between 'simple' and 'radical' mastectomies. Returning to the patient who had provided the starting point for the more general discussion, the surgeon told us,

> In this city, she'd have a simple mastectomy. In Edinburgh
> it's accepted that most units do a simple mastectomy ....

In both of these illustrations, then, appeal is made to 'Edinburgh' in recommending choices of treatment. 'The way things are done here' is a common enough appeal to local experience and ideology in most processes of socialisation, including socialisation into organisations and occupational groups. In the second example, the surgeon also draws attention to a further dimension of segmentation: 'most' units do a simple mastectomy, but it is not a categorical statement, and there is the possibility of differences in approach between units within the same city. The autonomy of practitioners allows for the development of different treatments of choice in different sectors of the same medical school.

Pharmacology is a topic where 'experience' is frequently drawn on in justifying or condemning the use of particular drugs or dosages. In the following field note, the physician refers to fashion and personal experience in decision-making in this field:

> The clinique then proceeded to a discussion of therapy.
> Dr. Mayo asked what drugs you would use to treat

rheumatoid arthritis. Tim Watson replied, 'Anti-inflammatory drugs - aspirin'. Dr. Mayo agreed that aspirin was still the best treatment, provided it relieves the pain sufficiently. He went on to comment on some other drugs which were, as he put it, 'in vogue', but which can produce unpleasant side effects.

Dr. Mayo went on to comment that one needs to monitor blood levels: in aspirin the upper limit of dosage was indicated by the patient experiencing 'ringing in the ears'. He pointed out that it was not always possible to get blood levels monitored, and so you have to 'use your own judgement'. And, he added, 'you need to use drugs you are used to'.

The empirical basis of some therapeutic procedures is frequently repeated, and contrasted with the claims of scientific knowledge. This is again illustrated in the following case, where the 'do or die' aspects of the treatment offered threw into relief the *practical* need for action, in contrast to the niceties of theoretical pharmacology.

Similarly, in the following extract, the physician refers to the possibilities of action by the *ad hoc* use of therapeutic techniques, as a possible departure from established procedure:

Dr. Rosen took us back to the teaching room, and told us that the patient we had just seen had multiple myeloma. He told us that there was no chance of a cure, but that they were about to embark on a course of palliative treatment. There were two drugs that they were going to use, both in fairly massive doses. He said that they were advised to treat patients of this sort for one month on the drugs, and one month off - to give the bone marrow a chance to recuperate. However, he added, they might find it better to administer the drugs one week on and one week off, or two weeks and two weeks respectively. 'One has to play it by ear', he concluded.

The warrant of experience is often referred to as a source of certainty or trust in the face of the vagaries of fashion and novelty. This too can be illustrated from the field of pharmaceuticals. Since the 'therapeutic revolution' in the 1930s, the number of different pharmaceutical preparations has increased exponentially (Norton, 1969). Doctors are being introduced to a vast range of medications for illnesses of all sorts. Many of the preparations that are taken up and widely used gain their popularity partly on the basis of 'fashion' (cf. Coleman *et al.*, 1966). Whilst 'fashion' and 'experience' can both be contrasted to 'science' they are also themselves contrasted. The dictates of fashion do not match up to carefully amassed personal experience in clinical practice.

The importance of experience and personal knowledge has been noted before. Becker and the other authors of *Boys in White* note the importance of experience for students and teachers alike. They identify a group perspective based upon this action, and they take the 'clinical experience perspective' to refer to 'actual experience in dealing with patients and disease ...'. As they comment, it is often used to contrast with 'theoretical' and 'scientific' knowledge:

> ... even though it substitutes for scientifically certified knowledge, it can be used to legitimate a choice of procedures for a patient's treatment and can even be used to rule out use of some procedures that have been scientifically established.

(Becker *et al.*, 1961, p.225)

This important place that is reserved for 'experience' has often been linked with constellation of factors referred to as 'uncertainty'. Freidson (1970) provides a classic formulation. He summarises the Kansas evidence, and then continues:

> ... the practitioner is very prone to emphasise the idea of indeterminacy or uncertainty, not the idea of regularity or of lawful, scientific behaviour. Whether or not that idea faithfully represents actual deficiencies in available knowledge or technique it does provide the practitioner with a psychological ground from which to justify his pragmatic emphasis on first hand experience.

Here Freidson emphasises uncertainty of knowledge, suggesting that personal knowledge and experience are to be contrasted with notions of regularity and predictability. He also tends to account for this at the level of the psychology of the individual practitioner. Fox (1957) takes a similar view in her discussion of 'training for uncertainty'. Like Freidson, she tends to treat it as a psychological problem that medical students need to come to terms with. I have already suggested one way in which such formulations may be inadequate. The idea of uncertainty or indetermination needs to be seen not simply as the outcome of individual psychology, but must also be seen in the context of professional segmentation, and as a reflection of the conditions of autonomy on the part of practitioners. Further, in both the formulations of the 'clinical mentality' referred to above, the theme of 'training for uncertainty' has been over-stressed. 'Training for dogmatism' has been almost entirely overlooked (Atkinson, 1984).

Dogmatism is by no means the opposite of personal knowledge; it is part and parcel of the same view of personal 'experience'. The clinician who appeals to his personal knowledge does so not by reference to his uncertainty, nor the uncertainty of his colleagues. Rather, he bases his actions and decisions on what is taken as a bedrock - the certainty - of direct experience. The appeal to experience is (*pace* Freidson) taken to provide knowledge of regularity and stability. The clinician operates in a state of personal certainty, in the sure warrant of his own personal experience. Hence the appeal to experience *is* taken to provide knowledge of regularity and stability; but this order is taken to be inherent in the phenomena, and open to the gaze, rather than residing in systems of theory and fashion. The clinic is therefore taken to provide the incontrovertible demonstrations of reality in direct perception of its regularities. The clinician is not therefore operating in a state of uncertainty, but rather operating on the sure warrant of her or his stock of experience. In this way, the students' exposure to this real world of medicine reproduces the warrant of personal knowledge.

9 Reproducing medicine

This book has been concerned with the social construction of reality in the context of one phase of medical education. While no claims can be entered as to the typicality of the particular, concrete details reported here, I do want to suggest that what I have reported reflects fundamental and general features of clinical medicine and medical education. The most important of these is the way in which a particular *version* of medical work and medical knowledge is reproduced through clinical instruction. This in turn reflects the basic premise of 'clinical experience' itself.

Clinical phases of training rest on the assumption that the trainee is to gain practical knowledge and experience through some form of exposure to, immersion in, and some sort of practice on real settings. Medical education provides the ideal type case of professional training of this sort; the designation 'clinical' has been transposed from medical settings to other occupational contexts. (It has, for instance, been applied to developments in legal education: see Rees, 1975.)

Throughout this short monograph, I have attempted to document how this clinical 'reality' is socially organised, achieved and managed. I have therefore provided a detailed account of how a particular sort of medical reality is produced and reproduced. No attempt has been made, therefore, to account for all aspects of undergraduate medical education, nor even to cover all aspects of everyday life among the students I observed and talked to. The focus of this book has been more limited than that, and it certainly does not aim to be a holistic ethnography. The theme of clinical experience has therefore been the dominant, organising theme of this book. In this conclusion I want briefly to consider the nature of that experience.

As I have shown, the medical reality to which the beginning student is exposed is by no means straightforward. There is nothing natural about such reality. Like any other it is a matter of social construction. What novitiate students are introduced to, then, is not the practical reality of some essential clinical medicine. Rather, they encounter the dramatic enactment of particular forms or versions of medical work. It is through that enactment that the potency of such a version of medicine is captured and reproduced. I hope I may have conveyed something of the vivid drama of that reproduction: as I suggested in Chapter 2 the medical students find themselves personally absorbed and intellectually seduced by this highly appealing form of work and understanding.

It is worth reminding the reader once again that the mind boggling methods of deduction expounded by the fictional Sherlock Holmes were taken by Conan Doyle from the real life methods of medical inference. (He must have enjoyed the irony that in his stories it was Dr. Watson, the medical man, who always proved too dense to follow the great detective's logic.) On numerous occasions during my fieldwork I was struck by the parallels between the Holmesian approach, and the displays of diagnostic acumen produced by the clinical teachers. I found myself identifying, at least tentatively, a style of teaching I labelled *thaumaturgical* (wonder working). The patients and medical students would find themselves recruited partly as audience, partly as stooges, partly as props in displays of clinical expertise and diagnostic skill. The effects of such displays, and of less dramatic styles of teaching too, is to produce vivid firsthand reconstructions of the logic and rationality of clinical medicine. It is as audience to these performances that the students gain their first clinical experiences.

There is something noteworthy here about the only photograph to accompany that classic ethnography, *Boys in White*. The picture appears on the original dust jacket. It shows seven male medical students, all looking remarkably similar in their white jackets and trousers. They are sitting in a steeply banked lecture theatre, of a kind used in medical schools from their earliest years to the present day. They all have their eyes fixed on something or someone at the front of the theatre; who or what it is we do not know. But this one photograph stands as a remarkable metonym for the nature of clinical education: the students as audience in a dramatic reconstruction, their clinical gaze fixed on their teachers and patients, and on the signs and symptoms they display, absorbed in the clinical world. The photograph from *Boys in White* does not reveal the object of the students' rapt attention: in that book Becker and his colleagues pay little attention to it. In this monograph I have attempted to follow their gaze, to follow the students' line of vision, and to devote my attention to the drama of clinical instruction.

Mock-ups and warrants for knowledge

Let me recapitulate what I take to be the main features of bedside teaching as cold medicine. Student work on patients is managed in such a way that it proceeds as if diagnostic work were starting afresh, although in most cases it is not. I suggest that the enactment of cold medicine is a *glossing device* (Garfinkel and Sacks, 1970): that is, a device for 'doing observable-reportable understanding', as they put it. In other words, bedside teaching practices are socially organised ways by which the actors produce something like a working model of medical diagnosis. Such a model makes observable and teachable the methods whereby physical examination and diagnosis are normally performed by competent members of the medical profession. Garfinkel and Sacks suggest something of the sort in their discussion of glossing practices which they refer to as 'mock-ups': they instance working models as an example:

> *Mock-Ups*. It is possible to buy a plastic engine that will tell something about how auto engines work. The plastic engine preserves certain properties of the auto engine. For example, it will show how the pistons move with respect to the crank shaft; how they are timed to a firing sequence, and so on .... Let us call that plastic engine an account of an observable state of affairs. We offer the following observations of that account's features. First, in the very way that it provides for an accurate representation of features in the actual situation, and in the very way it provides for an accurate representation of some relationships and some features in the observable situation, it also makes specifically and deliberately false provision of some of the *essential* features of that situation.
>
> (Garfinkel and Sacks, 1970, p.263)

That characterization of a mock-up encapsulates precisely the nature of 'cold medicine' as an account of real medicine. In the accomplishment of such accounting devices, we can see how bedside teaching makes 'accurate representations' of real medicine (in the methods of history taking, physical examination and diagnosis), and how this is possible since it makes 'specifically and deliberately false provision of some of the essential features'. That is, normal clinical methods can be employed insofar as the reality of previous clinical work is suppressed or held in abeyance for the duration of the teaching exercise. This feature of bedside interactions makes them controllable and manageable by the teaching clinician. The 'false provision' (that prior medical work may be discounted) means that the clinician can work the model and articulate the account.

The cold medicine mock-up can be illustrated and parallelled by considering teaching of the natural sciences in secondary schools (Atkinson and Delamont, 1977). The main feature of this has been an emphasis upon learning by 'discovery'. Rather than being the passive recipients of facts, delivered *ex cathedra* by the science teacher, and divorced from their immediate experience, school pupils should rather learn science by *doing* it. That is, they should discover science and scientific understanding by performing experiments themselves. The teacher's task became redefined as one of co-ordinating and guiding the pupils' own discoveries. Now it is by no means the case that the 'discovery' of phenomena in the natural world can proceed independently from the methods of inquiry employed in the discovery procedure. As Delamont (1973) has documented, the classroom practice of such mock-ups of the work of scientists requires a great deal of more or less covert stage management on the part of the teacher. The pupils' line of inquiry has to be curtailed by the science teacher if they are to look for the appropriate phenomena, arrive at the predicted observation, and hence discover the expected scientific facts.

In that sense the school science lesson and the bedside teaching period are similar, in that they both depend for their success on the teacher's acting as if the answer to the problem were not already known, but needed to be discovered afresh, thus parallelling real contexts where discovery (scientific or diagnostic) is in fact the outcome of scientists' or doctors' inquiries. In both cases, then, the nature of the mock-up depends upon the discovery of appropriate conclusions, by the use of appropriate methods of inquiry ('experiments' or 'history taking and physical examination'). In my discussion of bedside teaching I have explored how 'cold medicine' provides occasion for the reproduction of clinical and diagnostic methods. In other words, how the practices of bedside instruction provide concrete demonstrations of the warranted nature of clinical knowledge.

We also need to consider how the 'facts of the case' are determined and legitimated by reference to the procedural rules of correct and methodical inquiry. When we speak of ascertaining the facts we assign a special status to certain sorts of accounts and propositions, as opposed to 'opinions', 'beliefs', 'guesses' and so on; by implication these latter are not granted the same warrant as well researched, fully documented, correctly retrieved facts. The status of such facts is not something which is inherent in the accounts of them - but rather resides in the procedures and rules that are used to establish and validate the knowledge. This is expressed by McHugh (1970):

> Nothing - no object, event, or circumstance - determines its own status as truth, either to the scientist or to science .... An event is transformed into the truth only by the application of a canon of procedure, a canon that truth-seekers use and analysts must formulate as providing the possibility of agreement.

The place of such methodic procedures in the determination of facts is highlighted in Kuhn's analysis of scientific revolutions (Kuhn, 1970). For Kuhn, it is the scientific 'paradigm' which provides the ground rules for scientists' consensus over appropriate topics for inquiry, appropriate methods and the sort of answers that might reasonably be expected. As Kuhn himself put it, the paradigms

> provide scientists not only with a map but also with the directions for map-making. In learning a paradigm the scientist acquires theory, methods, and standards together, usually in an inextricable mixture.

Kuhn's analysis of 'normal' and 'revolutionary' phases in scientific research and discovery draws attention to the fact that the practice of scientific inquiry is inescapably a *social* activity, insofar as it depends upon the organised consensus of those engaged in science and on their shared methods for the production of scientific knowledge.

The problem of ascertaining the warranting of 'facts of the case' is by no means confined to natural scientists. It appears as a practical problem in a wide range of everyday work. This is well documented by Zimmerman (1966, 1974) in his study of case workers in a social welfare agency. It was a routine problem for the case workers that they should establish whether applicants are entitled to the money and assistance which they claim. Applicants need to demonstrate need, and the agency workers must determine their eligibility. There is, therefore, a crucial distinction between the claimant's story and the facts. For a story to become transferred into a factual account, the case worker must check and validate the reliability of the claimant's account. One important aspect of this process is the way in which case workers rely on documentary evidence. Yet in establishing documentary evidence, 'any old piece of paper' will not do and only official documents will suffice. Such documents are taken to guarantee that the recorded facts have themselves been investigated, processed and recorded in a 'correct' and methodic manner. Bureaucracies and large-scale organisations are taken to operate in methodic ways which the case workers recognise as competent in producing facts and evidence.

In the same way, the case worker herself assembles documents on the applicant - producing a case which itself records the case worker's 'investigative stance' of scepticism and methodic inquiry. Thus the case worker assembles the 'facts of the case' in accordance with the legitimate rules of procedures of the bureaucracy, and bases her case on evidence provided by comparable bureaucracies employing equivalent methods of inquiry and documentation. Zimmerman thus points out how workers, whose task it is to produce orderly factual accounts, depend upon the demonstrable, rational and methodic ways in which their accounts have been assembled.

A similar perspective is provided by Smith (1973) in her discussion of the production of documentary reality, which she describes as 'constituted in those socially organised practices of reporting and accounting, which mediate our relation to "what really happens"'. Smith emphasises how the fact is not what happened in its raw or uninterpreted state. Factual status resides in the way 'what happened' has been worked up into an account of which itself provides for a factual reading and understanding. The nature of 'factual' accounts, however, allows the reader or hearer to treat them in such a way as to discount their social nature: the organisation of the account is itself transparent. In this context Smith draws a parallel between the social production of facts and the production of commodities. Marx wrote:

> A commodity is ... a mysterious thing, simply because in it the social character of man's labour appears to them as an objective character stamped upon the product of that labour.
>
> (Marx, 1954, p.77)

Although such products are created by human labour, nevertheless they confront their producers as alien objects; the relations between social actors take on a nature of relations between things. In much the same way, Smith argues, facts are equally 'mysterious'. They are outcomes of the socially organised ways of dealing with events. Yet they do not appear to be socially produced by actors engaged in practical action. On the contrary, we normally employ the notions of 'opinion', 'belief', 'ideology' and 'bias' to locate the social nature of such knowledge; the language of 'fact' excludes the mediation of the social basis of knowledge production.

I wish to consider the practices of bedside teaching in the light of the production of factual knowledge. Cold medicine is a device whereby the rational and methodic nature of clinical investigation and the retrieval of the facts of the case are produced and reproduced. There is a dialectical relationship between facts and the socially legitimated methods for their discovery and testing. The methodic nature of their production is a warrant for the correctness of the facts of the case. At the same time, it is the reliable discovery of such facts that further furnishes a warrant for the methods of inquiry. I take it that this is the force of Kuhn's notion of normal science, conducted in accordance with a paradigm. The paradigm provides approved topics and appropriate research procedures; the successful accomplishment of such procedures and the findings that are generated in turn serve to reinforce the value of the paradigm.

Factual accounts are 'reflexive' (Garfinkel, 1967). That is, accounts are themselves constitutive of the affairs they describe. As Filmer (1972) paraphrases Garfinkel:

> rules ... are only established as such by their ability to organize the settings of practical, everyday, commensense actions - an ability which is proven in organising these actions.

In the medical context, therefore, the facts of a diagnosis are guaranteed by the rules and procedures of clinical inquiry which establish them: by the same token, these procedures are validated insofar as they generate reproduceable and reportable diagnoses.

Displays of the rational nature of such socially warranted methods are an important ingredient in a novice's learning of how to become a competent investigator of facts. Zimmerman (1974) refers to this in his discussion of welfare agency workers. Those who were new in the job were instructed by the old hands in the correct application of the rules of investigative procedure. It was part of their practical training that they should adopt a sufficiently sceptical attitude towards applicants' stories, and address the relevant criteria to establish (or disprove) the factual basis of such claims. This is assured by their search for appropriate documentary evidence, as they inspect the methods whereby such evidence is produced and assembled.

In the same way, the performance of clinical teaching depends upon concrete displays of the efficacy of the investigative stance and procedures of the competent clinician. It is in this light, therefore, that one must consider the reconstruction of the patient's case in the course of the bedside encounter.

The practice of guided discovery in students' diagnoses (as in school science) is a version of what Bernstein referred to as 'invisible pedagogy' (Bernstein, 1975). The distinction between visible and invisible pedagogies rests on the manner in which cultural transmission and reproduction are accomplished: 'The more implicit the manner of transmission ... the more invisible the pedagogy'. Bernstein's arguments are formulated primarily in connection with varieties of preschool and infant education, but they can be extended to many other settings. One of the essential characteristics of invisible pedagogy, as identified by Bernstein, is that 'ideally, the teacher arranges the *context* which the child is expected to rearrange and explore'. This facet of invisible pedagogy can likewise be seen in the contrivances of bedside teaching, which also depend upon the student's exploration of a largely prearranged and stage-managed field of experience.

It is in the nature of invisible pedagogies that the social mechanisms of knowledge transmission should not themselves be explicit. Hence the organisation and construction of legitimated knowledge pass for an organisation that is inherent in phenomena of the real world under exploration and investigation. The invisible pedagogy of bedside teaching practices provide a mechanism for the affirmation of the preconstituted nature of illness as an ontological entity, while the social production of disease categories remains invisible.

Hence the warrant for the clinical is constantly reaffirmed through the organised practices of bedside instruction. As Armstrong (1980) puts it:

> In the clinical years emphasis is placed on how to gain knowledge (through the process of diagnosis) as against learning particular items of knowledge. This stress on ways of creating knowledge emphasises the legitimacy of the clinical gaze and its inherent epistemology. Diagnosis is the apotheosis of such method, and whether this skill is described as 'clinical sense', 'clinical ability' or the 'art of diagnosis' the doctor is ranked according to his facility with the technique.

196

In thus warranting the epistemology of clinical knowledge, bedside instruction affirms the primacy of personal experience. It is at once the means of imparting, and the charter for, the 'clinical mentality' which Freidson (1970, p. 170) captured so well:

> In having to rely so heavily upon his personal, clinical experience with concrete, individual cases...the practitioner comes essentially to rely on the authority of his own senses, independently of the general authority of tradition or science. After all, he can only act on the basis of what he himself experiences, and if his own activity seems to get results, or at least no untoward results, he is resistant to changing it on the basis of statistical or abstract considerations. He is likely to need to see or feel the case himself.

Hence the clinician becomes committed to 'his faith, his pragmatism, his subjectivism', what Freidson also calls 'a rather thoroughgoing particularism, a kind of ontological and epistemological individualism'.

This faith in the primacy of firsthand perception and personal experience leads to the clinician's certainty, in that his or her knowledge and action is unassailably warranted by the touchstone of experience. This is not to deny, of course, that medical practitioners take account of other forms and sources of information: rather, that personal knowledge is granted a special privilege. The rationale for this privilege may be conveyed by paraphrasing Foucault's comments on the clinical gaze (cf. Foucault, 1973, p. 54): the patient's bedside has always been a place of constant, stable experience, in contrast to theories and systems, which have been in perpetual change and have masked beneath their speculation the purity of clinical evidence. The gaze thus furnishes the bedrock of certainty on which the practitioner relies.

Throughout this monograph I have attempted to address two recurring and closely linked themes. They are: the performative aspects of medical instruction, and the social forms through which clinical medicine is reproduced. In the years since the fieldwork was completed and the first edition of this ethnography was published, much has changed in the organization of British medical education. Widespread curricular reform has taken place, largely in response to the *Tomorrow's Doctors* reforms promulgated by the UK General Medical Council. It would be very easy to dismiss the empirical basis of the ethnography as holding historical interest only - though perhaps an interesting historical document, capturing the late flowering of a disappearing tradition of clinical instruction. To do so, however, would be to miss extraordinary continuities in the social organization of medical work and the social production of medical knowledge. As I indicated in Chapter 1, there is an unbroken tradition of clinical instruction that links Edinburgh with Leyden and the direct influence of Boerhaave (Rosner, 1991). Notwithstanding the very great changes that have affected the content and organization of medicine - the development of physical diagnosis, the introduction of aseptic surgery and anaesthesia, or the therapeutic revolution - the oral performance of medicine reflects many continuities from that early modern period. The dramatic enactment of medicine on the wards and in the clinical lecture, the oral tradition of recitation and the narrative formats of case presentations all reflect the *longue durée* of clinical forms. To borrow and extend (but not, I think, distort) Strong's telling title, the ceremonial order of the clinic (Strong, 1979) is a powerful mechanism through which the coherence and stability of the profession of medicine are sustained.

Elsewhere (Atkinson, 1989) I have commented on the remarkable archival material that survives from the early years of this century in the United States. The teaching clinics of a physician were recorded and transcibed by a stenographer (Davenport, 1987). The content of the medicine is not, of course, identical with that of the present: the diseases with which patients present differ in their incidence, and the available treatments differ greatly. But the forms of discourse are remarkably similar to those I documented in the Edinburgh medical school over half a century later. The continuity is quite striking, despite the distances of space and time. The production of definitions of clinical entities, the appeal to the clinician's experience, and the distinctive registers of clinical instruction are all recognisable. Indeed, were it not for the specific differences in clinical terminology, one would be hard pressed to find significant differences from the clinical discourse of the late twentieth century.

The performance of clinical medicine is most immediately visible through its overtly theatrical manifestations. Clinical medicine is rendered spectacular through the more florid displays of large-scale lectures and presentations. Its dramaturgical aspects are, in addition, enacted on a smaller scale and more intimately, in the daily work of reality-construction on the wards and in the clinics. The clinical teacher performs as a thaumaturge, conjuring wonders out of the signs and symptoms of bedside instruction. Through this work of dramatization, the patient's body is rendered meaningful. The significance - indeed, the work of signifying - of the physical examination was not established once and for all in the great teaching hospitals of Paris, Vienna and in Edinburgh itself. It is reaffirmed and rediscovered every day through the encounters between clinicians and their students. The ceremonial progress of the round is one of the circuits of discourse through which the clinic is organized (cf. Atkinson, 1995; Fox, 1992) and through which its interactional order is sustained. It is the site of an oral culture and of the inter-generational transmission of knowledge.

The medicine of the ward and of the bedside is itself an ancient one. For all the technical changes in medicine, the fragmentation of specialties and the proliferation of medical representations, it remains a clinical medicine rooted in signs and symptoms. As I have tried to document through the ethnographic detail of this monograph, the recapitulations and displays of diagnostic inference are powerful. The patient's history and the patient's body are made to yield up the *differentia specifica* of clinical entities. The medical student's acquisition of knowledge and experience recapitulate the classical methods of physical examination and diagnosis, while classical nosographies are also recapitulated. We glimpse repeatedly through the ethnography of bedside teaching how students learn to map the terrain of disease. Classic cases and pathognomic signs encode the array of diseases and their characteristic trajectories. Such clinical instruction implicitly claims to reveal a world of categorical diseases or clinical entities. It is a nosography of recognition and of naming practices. It is a clinical practice of lists, differences and types. Evident most clearly in the teaching of internal medicine, it is equally evident in surgery, with its repeated stress on discrete lesions, single anatomical sites, and its short time-scale.

This, then, is a medicine of clinical entities. It follows a natural history of diseases and is grounded in bedside interaction. Its distinctive forms of social interaction form the immediate social context in which that medical culture is enacted. The focused huddle that forms and re-forms in the physical space by the patient's bed furnishes the participants and the audience for the dramaturgy of the clinic. It is a locus for the privileged perceptions of the clinical gaze. It is not, of course, the only setting of medical education, and it is not the only form of medicine that may be acquired. It is, none the less, fundamental to the reproduction of a pervasive and persistent strand of medical culture.

Bibliography

Armstrong, D. (1980) Health care and the structure of medical education, in Noack, H. (ed.) *Medical Education and Primary Health Care*. London: Croom Helm.

Atkinson, P.A. (1971) Kind hearts and curettes, *New Society*, 27 July, pp.178-90.

Atkinson, P.A. (1973) Worlds apart: learning environments in medicine and surgery, *British Journal of Medical Education*, 7, 218-24.

Atkinson, P.A. (1974) 'Centre' and 'periphery': further analysis of learning environments in the Edinburgh medical school, *British Journal of Medical Education*, 8, 234-40.

Atkinson, P.A. (1976) *The Clinical Experience: An Ethnography of Medical Education*, unpublished Ph.D. thesis, University of Edinburgh.

Atkinson, P.A. (1977a) Professional segmentation and students' experience in a Scottish medical school, *Scottish Journal of Sociology*, 2, 71-85.

Atkinson, P.A. (1977b) Becoming a hypochondriac, in G. Horobin and A. Davis (eds) *Medical Encounters*. London: Croom Helm.

Atkinson, P.A. (1983) The reproduction of professional community, in Dingwall, R. and Lewis, P. (eds) *The Sociology of the Professions: Lawyers, Doctors and Others*. London: Macmillan.

Atkinson, P.A. (1984) Training for certainty, *Social Science and Medicine*, 19, 949-56.

Atkinson, P.A. (1984) Wards and deeds: taking knowledge and control seriously, in Burgess, R.G. (ed.) *The Research Process in Educational Settings:Ten Case Studies*. Lewes: Falmer.

Atkinson, P.A. (1989) Voices from the past, *Sociology of Health and Illness*, 11, 78-82.

Atkinson, P.A. (1995) *Medical Talk and Medical Work*. London: Sage.

Atkinson, P.A. (1996) *Sociological Readings and Re-Readings.* Aldershot: Avebury.

Atkinson, P.A. and Delamont S. (1977) Mock-ups and cock-ups: the stage-mangement of guided discovery instruction, in Woods P. and Hammersley, M. (eds) *School Experience.* London: Croom Helm.

Atkinson P.A., Reid, M.E. and Sheldrake, P.F. (1977) Medical mystique, *Sociology of Work and Occupations*, 4, 243-80.

Becker, H.S. and Geer, B. (1958) The fate of idealism in medical school, *American Sociological Review*, 23, 50-66.

Becker, H.S. and Geer, B. (1960) Latent culture: a note on the theory of latent social roles, *Administrative Science Quarterly*, 5, 304-13.

Becker, H.S. Geer, B., Hughes, E.C. and Strauss, A.L. (1961) *Boys in White: Student Culture in Medical School.* Chicago: University of Chicago Press.

Berger, P. and Luckmann, T. (1967) *The Social Construction of Reality.* London: Allen Lane.

Bernstein, B. (1975) Class pedagogies: visible and invisible, in *Class, Codes and Control.* Vol.3. London: Routledge and Kegan Paul.

Bucher, R. and Stelling, J.G. (1977) *Becoming Professional.* Beverly Hills: Sage.

Cartwright, A. (1964) *Human Relations and Hospital Care.* London: Routledge and Kegan Paul.

Coffey, A.J., Holbrook, B. and Atkinson, P.A. (1996) Qualitative data analysis: technologies and representations, *Sociological Research Online*, 1, 1, < www.socresonline.ac.uk >

Coleman, J., Katz, E. and Menzel, H. (1966) *Medical Innovation: A Diffusion Study.* Indianapolis: Bobbs-Merrill.

Comrie, J.D. (1932) *History of Scottish Medicine* (2 vols.). London: Balliere, Tindall and Cox.

Crooks, J. (1974) Clinical Teaching in the Medical Curriculum of the University of Dundee, in *Curriculum Changes in United Kingdom Medical Schools.* Dundee: Association for the Study of Medical Education, Dundee.

Davenport, H.W. (1987) *Doctor Dock: Teaching and Learning Medicine at the Turn of the Century.* New Brunswick: Rutgers University Press.

Davis, F. (1959) The cab-driver and his fare: facets of a fleeting relationship, *American Journal of Sociology*, 65, 158-65.

Davis F. (1960) Comment on "Initial interaction of newcomers in Alcoholics Anonymous", *Social Problems*, 8, 364-65.

Davis, F. (1961) Deviance disavowal: the management of strained interaction by the visibly handicapped, *Social Problems*, 9, 120-32.

Davis, F. (1963) *Passage Through Crisis*. Indianapolis: Bobbs-Merrill.

Davis, F. (1968) Professional socialization as subjective experience: the process of doctrinal conversation among student nurses, in Becker, H.S. *et al.* (eds) *Institutions and the* Person. Chicago: Aldine.

Delamont, K.S. (1973) *Academic Conformity Observed: Studies in the Classroom*, unpublished Ph.D thesis, University of Edinburgh.

DelVecchio Good, M-J. (1995) *American Medicine: The Quest for Competence*. Berkeley: University of California Press.

Dingwall, R. (1977) *The Social Organisation of Health Visitor Training*. London: Croom Helm.

Dowling, H.F. and Cotsonas, N.H. (1964) The training of the physician: attitudes toward patients of full-time and practising instructors as revealed in student questionnaires, *New England Journal of Medicine*, 271, 716-18.

Eastwood, M. (1972) The Edinburgh of 1821, *Synapse*, 21, 11-14.

Ellis, J.R. (1975) Should the medical course be shortened? in *Curriculum Changes in United Kingdom Medical Schools*. Dundee: Association for the Study of Medical Education.

Emerson, J.P. (1970) Behavior in private places: sustaining definitions of reality in gynaecological examinations, in Dreitzel, H.P. (ed.) *Recent Sociology, No.2: Patterns of Communicative Behaviour*. London: Collier-Macmillan.

Emerson, R.M. and Pollner, M. (1978) Politics and practices of psychiatric case selection, *Sociology of Work and Occupations*, 5, 75-96.

Eron, L.D. (1955) Effect of medical education on medical students' attitudes, *Journal of Medical Education*, 30, 559-66.

Fabian, J. (1983) *Time and The Other: How Anthropology Makes Its Object*. New York, Columbia University Press.

Ferris, P. (1967) *The Doctors*. Harmondsworth: Penguin.

Filmer, P. (1972) On Harold Garfinkel's ethnomethodology, in Filmer, P., Phillipson, M., Silverman, D., and Walsh, D., *New Directions in Sociological Theory*. London: Collier-Macmillan.

Flexner, A. (1925) *Medical Education, A Comparative Study*. New York: Macmillan.

Foucault, M. (1973) *The Birth of the Clinic*. London: Tavistock.

Fox, N.J. (1992) *The Social Meaning of Surgery*. Milton Keynes: Open University Press.

Fox, R. (1957) Training for uncertainty, in Merton, R.K., Reader, G. and Kendall, P.L (eds) *The Student Physician*. Cambridge, Mass.: Harvard University Press.

Fox, R. (1959) *Experiment Perilous*. Glencoe: Free Press.

Freidson, E. (1970) *Profession of Medicine*. New York: Dodd Mead.

Garfinkel, H. (1967) *Studies in Ethnomethodology*. Englewood Cliffs: Prentice-Hall.

Garfinkel, H. and Sacks H. (1970) On formal structures of practical actions, in McKinney, J.C. and Tiryakian, E.A. (eds) *Theoretical Sociology: Perspectives and Developments*. New York: Appleton-Century-Crofts.

Geer, B. (1964) First days in the field, in Hammond, P. (ed.) *Sociologists at Work*. New York: Basic Books.

Geer, B., Haas, J., Vona, C.V., Miller, S.J., Woods, C. and Becker, H.S. (1968) Learning the ropes: situational learning in four occupational training programs, in Deutscher, I. and Thompson, E.J. (eds) *Among the People*. New York: Basic Books.

Glaser, B. and Strauss, A.L. (1964) Awareness contexts and social interaction, *American Sociological Review*, 29, 669-79.

Glaser, B. and Strauss, A.L. (1965) *Awareness of Dying*. Chicago: Aldine.

Goffman, E. (1961) *Encounters: Two Studies in the Sociology of Interaction*. Indianapolis: Bobbs-Merrill.

Goffman, E. (1968) *Asylums*. Harmondsworth: Penguin.

Goffman, E. (1971) *The Presentation of Self in Everyday Life*. Harmondsworth: Penguin.

Goffman, E. (1972) *Relations in Public*. Harmondsworth: Penguin.

Gold, R.L. (1958) Roles in sociological fieldwork, *Social Forces*, 36, 217-23.

Haas, J. and Shaffir, W. (1977) The professionalization of medical students: developing competence and a cloak of competence, *Symbolic Interaction*, 71-88.

Hall, O. (1948) The stages of a medical career, *American Journal of Sociology*, 53, 327-36.

Hughes, E.C. (1958) *Men and Their Work*. Glencoe: Free Press.

Humphreys, L. (1970) *Tearoom Trade*. Chicago: Aldine.

Jamous, H. and Peloille, B. (1970) Professions or self-perpetuating system? Changes in the French university-hospital system, in

Jackson, J.A. (ed.) *Professions and Professionalization*. Cambridge: Cambridge University Press.

Kuhn, T.S. (1970) *The Structure of Scientific Revolutions*. Chicago: University of Chicago Press.

Lief, H.I. and Fox, R.C. (1963) Training for 'detached concern' in medical students, in Lief, H.I. *et al.* (eds) *The Psychological Basis of Medical Practice*. New York: Harper and Row.

Lofland, J. (1971) *Analyzing Social Settings*. Belmont: Wadsworth.

Lofland, J.F. and Lejeune, R.A. (1960) Initial interaction of newcomers in Alcoholics Anonymous, *Social Problems*, 8, 102-111.

MacCannell, D. (1977) *The Tourist*. London: Macmillan.

McHugh, P. (1970) The failure of positivism, in Douglas, J. (ed.) *Understanding Everyday Life*. London: Routledge and Kegan Paul.

Manning, P. (1971) Talking and becoming: a view of organizational socialization, in Douglas, J. (ed.) *Understanding Everyday Life*. London: Routledge and Kegan Paul.

Marx, K. (1954) *Capital: A Critical Analysis of Capitalist Production*. Moscow: Foreign Languages Publishing House.

Mechanic, D. (1968) *Medical Sociology*. New York: Free Press.

Merton, R.K., Reader, G. and Kendall, P.L. (eds) (1957) *The Student Physician*. Cambridge, Mass.: Harvard University Press.

Miller, S.J. (1970) *Prescription for Leadership: Training for the Medical Elite*. Chicago: Aldine.

Mills, C.W. (1940) Situated actions and vocabularies of motive, *American Sociological Review*, 5, 439-52.

Newman, C. (1957) *The Evolution of Medical Education in the Nineteenth Century*. London: Oxford University Press.

Norton, A. (1969) *Drugs, Science and Society*. London: Hodder and Stoughton.

Olesen, V. and Whittaker, E. (1968) *The Silent Dialogue: The Social Psychology of Professional Socialisation*. San Fransisco: Jossey-Bass.

Olesen, V. and Whittaker, E. (1970) Critical notes on sociological studies of professional socialisation, in Jackson, J.A. (ed.) *Professions and Professionalisation*. Cambridge: Cambridge University Press.

Rees, W. (1975) Clinical legal education: an analysis of the University of Kent model, *The Law Teacher*, 9, 125-40.

Rosenberg, P. (1969) The freshman medical student circa 1968-69: a dynamic analysis, paper presented to the Eighth Annual Conference on Research in Medical Education.

204

Rosner, L. (1991) *Medical Education in the Age of Improvement*. Edinburgh: Edinburgh University Press.

Roth, J. (1961) Comments on 'secret observation', *Social Problems*, 9, 283-84.

Roth, J. (1963) *Timetables*. Indianapolis: Bobbs-Merrill.

Roth, J. (1974) Professionalism: the sociologist's decoy, *Sociology of Work and Occupations*, 1, 6-23.

Royal Commission on Medical Education (1968) *Report 1965-68* Cmnd. 3569. London: HMSO (The Todd Report).

Schatzman, L. and Strauss, A.L. (1973) *Field Research*. Englewood Cliffs: Prentice-Hall.

Schutz, A. (1964) *Collected Papers, Vol. 2*, The Hague: Martinus Nijhoff.

Shuval, J. (1975) From 'boy' to 'colleague': processes of role transformation in professional socialization, *Social Science and Medicine*, 9, 413-20.

Silverman, D. (1975) *Reading Castaneda: A Prologue to the Social Sciences*. London: Routledge and Kegan Paul.

Smith, D. (1973) The social construction of documentary reality, paper presented at the meeting of the Canadian Sociological and Anthropological Association, Queens University, Kingston, Ontario.

Stimson, G. and Webb, B. (1975) *Going to See the Doctor*. London: Routledge and Kegan Paul.

Stoddart, K. (1974) Pinched: notes on the ethnographer's location of argot, in Turner, R. (ed.) *Ethnomethodology*. Harmondsworth: Penguin.

Stokes, J.F. (1974) *The Clinical Examination*. Dundee: Association for the Study of Medical Education.

Strauss, A.L., Schatzman, L., Ehrlich, D., Bucher, R. and Sabshin, M. (1963) The hospital and its negotiated order, in Freidson, E. (ed.) *The Hospital in Modern Society*. Glencoe: Free Press.

Strong, P.M. (1979) *The Ceremonial Order of the Clinic*. London: Routledge and Kegan Paul.

Stubbs, M. (1975) Teaching and talking: a sociolinguistic approach to classroom interaction, in Chanan, G. and Delamont, S. (eds) *Frontiers of Classroom Research*. Slough: National Foundation for Educational Research.

Sudnow, D. (1965) Normal crimes, *Social Problems*, 12, 255-76.

Sudnow, D. (1967) *Passing On: The Social Organization of Dying*. Englewood Cliffs: Prentice-Hall.

Templeton, B., (1964) Hazards of teaching adult medicine at the bedside (Abstract), *Journal of Medical Education*, 42, 278.

Turner, R. (1972) Some formal properties of therapy talk, in Sudnow, D. (ed.) *Studies in Social Interaction*. Glencoe: Free Press.

Van Gennep, A. (1960) *The Rites of Passage*. Chicago: University of Chicago Press.

Wardwell, W.I. (1963) Limited, marginal and quasi-practitioners, in Freeman, H.E., Levine, S. and Reeder, L.G. (eds) *Handbook of Medical Sociology*. Englewood Cliffs: Prentice-Hall.

Weaver, A. and Atkinson, P.A. (1994) *Microcomputing Strategies for Qualitative Data Analysis*. Aldershot: Avebury.

Wieder, L. (1974) *Language and Social Reality: The Case of Telling the Convict Code*. The Hague: Mouton.

Woods, P. (1975) Showing them up in secondary school, in G. Chanan and S. Delamont (eds) *Frontiers of Classroom Research*. Slough: National Foundation for Educational Research.

Zimmerman, D.H. (1966) *Paper Work and People Work: A Study of a Public Assistance Agency*, unpublished PhD dissertation, University of California, Los Angeles.

Zimmerman, D.H. (1970) The practicalities of rule use, in Douglas, J. (ed.) *Understanding Everyday Life*. London: Routledge and Kegan Paul.

Zimmerman, D.H. (1974) Facts as a practical accomplishment, in Turner, R. (ed.) *Ethnomethodology*. Harmondsworth: Penguin.